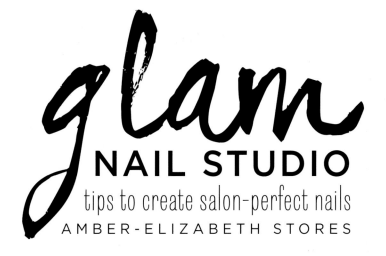

glam
NAIL STUDIO
tips to create salon-perfect nails
AMBER-ELIZABETH STORES

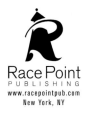

Race Point
PUBLISHING
www.racepointpub.com
New York, NY

Race Point
PUBLISHING

A division of Book Sales, Inc.
276 Fifth Avenue Suite 206
New York, New York 10001

RACE POINT PUBLISHING and the distinctive
Race Point Publishing logo are trademarks of Book Sales, Inc.

AUTHOR: Amber Elizabeth Stores
EDITOR: Tracy Sway Hofstatter
DESIGNER: Susan Van Horn
PHOTOGRAPHER: Tim Palin Creative

ISBN: 978-1-937994-24-2

Printed in China

2 4 6 8 10 9 7 5 3 1

www.racepointpub.com

To my mother Whendy, my father Bill, and my son Christian for being my driving force and my reason.

✳

To my best friends Serena Minton and Ravi Lambert for the constant support that comes through actions as well as words.

✳

To the team whose hard work, creativity, patience, and dedication turned this book from a dream to a reality.

✳

And lastly, to all the women and men who seek to make the world a more glamorous place along with me.

SPECIAL THANKS TO OUR HAND MODELS

Emma Cohen
Jamella David
Britni Dorset-Aleong
Brianna Fordham
Brittany Groth

Natalie Kathleen
Priya Mosher
Christina Nguyen
Jasmine Niang
Emilie Seaman

Megan Shelby
Athena Stuebe
Sienna Stuebe
Jill Futerman Sullivan
Lily Wass

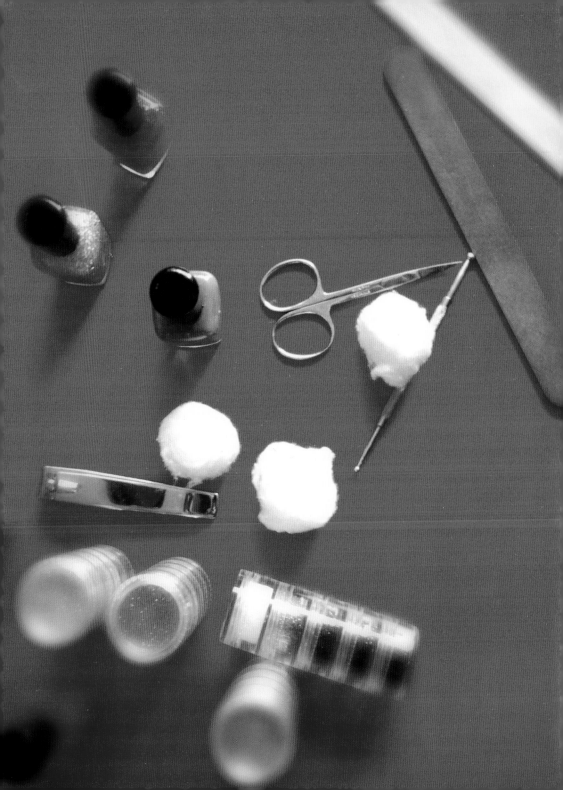

✳ contents ✳

INTRODUCTION......9

Chapter 1
HAND AND NAIL BASICS......11

Chapter 2
USING THE RIGHT TOOLS......25

Chapter 3
NAIL POLISH AND ENHANCEMENTS......35

Chapter 4
MANICURES AND PEDICURES......67

Chapter 5
BEYOND THE BASICS......91

Chapter 6
NAIL ART......111

Dotted Frames 114
Flowers 116
Pretty Polka Dots 118
Jackson Pollock 120
Leopard Print 122
Camouflage 124
Ombré 126
Pearly Net 128
Galaxy 130
Vintage Jewels 132
Neon Sparkle 134
Modern French 136
Rainbow Bright 138
Crosshatch 140
Zebra Print 142
Lightning Bolt 144
Zigzag Swag 146

Hearts 148
Bow 150
Music notes 152
Checkered Print 154
Argyle 156
Plaid 158
Geometric Shapes 160
Stars and Stripes 162
Tribal 164
Art Deco 166
Rock Star 168
Nautical 170
Smiley Face 172
Paris is for Lovers 174
Up in Flames 176
Vintage Lace 178
Frosted Cupcake 180

Puzzle 182
Springtime Flowers 184
Summer Fun 186
Autumn Leaves 188
Let it Snow 190
Pow! 192
Beauty Queen 194
Pucker Up 196
Tootie Fruity 198
Crystal Flowers 200
Court Jester 202
Dark Crystal 204
Modern Pop 206
Retro Cartoon 208
Haute Couture 210
Gilded City 212

MORE DIY INSPIRATION......214

GLOSSARY......219

introduction

An old proverb said,
"The nails are the windows to the soul."

No, wait—those are the eyes.

Well, if the eyes are the windows to the soul, the nails are the windows to the personality. Your nails are the ultimate way to express yourself! It's easy to tell if a gal is a rocker chick, girly girl, corporate diva, or busy bee with just a quick glance at her tips. Perfectly dressed nails exude confidence and swag, while half-bitten, chewed-up, dirty fingertips send out another message. (Sad, but true.)

Now, more than ever, nail care has blown up to become an essential part of your grooming routine. When you add nail art to your style, you have the perfect opportunity to let your imagination and self-expression run wild.

With just a quick flick of a polish brush, you can stay trendy and en vogue for days. Nail art has more staying power than that perfect smoky eye you begrudgingly have to wash off at the end of the night. Yet nails don't require the same kind of commitment as the edgy, eccentric haircut you grow tired of after only a week. Well-dressed nails pull your look together with minimal effort, and make a statement about who you are and what matters to you.

Really, no matter how you roll, being well groomed implies that you're focused, put-together, and ready to bring your "A-game" . . . from tip to toes!

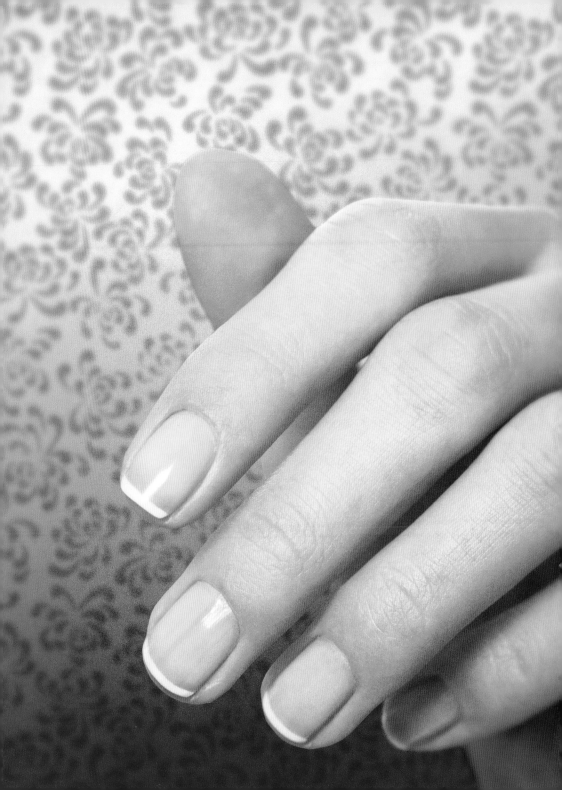

CHAPTER ONE

hand and nail basics

When an admirer asks to get a closer look

at your super-stylin' nails, you proudly present those color-covered tips. But those pops of color on your fingertips are just the tip—one of the numerous parts that make up the whole of your fingernails. We are all familiar with the part that we can easily see, but it's helpful to review the entire nature and purpose of these 20 complex little structures. After all, to safely and easily turn out an eye-popping manicure without damage, we must first examine the blueprint of our nail. Along the way, we'll reveal some interesting data. For instance, did you know that nails are mainly made up of the same bodily ingredients as hair and skin—a protein called keratin? And that fact is just the tip of the iceberg. Let's try to wrap our brains around the anatomy of these tiny little canvases before we break out the paint.

✳ STRUCTURE AND COMPOSITION OF THE NAIL

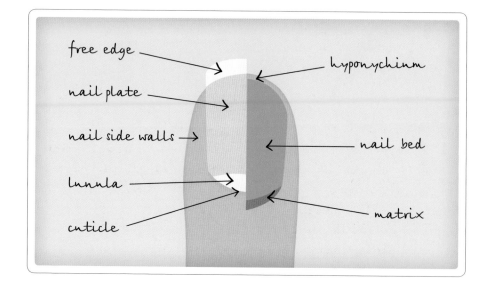

The Cuticle

The cuticle is the least-loved part of the nail. It is formed of semi-transparent dead tissues attached to the base of the nail plate. The cuticle is constantly pushed, cut, and overworked, but it does an important job and has good reason for being there. Think of the cuticle as a security guard protecting a doorway; it seals the space between the nail plate and your skin, preventing germs, bacteria, and cooties from getting into your bod and causing a ruckus.

The cuticle guards more than just the health of your hands and nails; it protects your entire body from unwanted germs. If you find yourself prone to colds and flus, you may want to think about how you cut and care for your cuticles.

The Free Edge

The free edge is the portion of the nail plate that extends past the nail bed. As the nail plate grows, your free edge is formed and slowly inches past your fingertips, waiting to be filed, cut, or (the worst thing ever) bitten. The free edge is the extension of the nail plate and also the hardest part of the nail. Its purpose is to protect the tips of your fingers.

The Hyponychium
(hy-poh-NIK-ee-um)
Think of the hyponychium as another cuticle under the nail plate. It's the seal located under the free edge, and it forms the curved line that shows through the nail plate. The hyponychium serves the same purpose as the cuticle, guarding your body from uninvited cooties. This seal also hurts like crazy when detached.

The Lunula
The lunula is the half-moon shape located at the bottom of the nail near the cuticle. The lighter color indicates the transition stage of the nail from live to dead. Don't worry if you can't find yours; not everyone has visible lunulas.

The Matrix
The matrix is the only living part of the nail. It's the place where nail growth originates, and where new nail cells are formed. Any damage to the matrix is irreparable.

The Nail Bed
Think of the nail bed as the comfy cushion for the nail plate. The nail bed is composed of living tissues right underneath the nail plate, where all of the blood vessels and nerves live. These tissues deliver the nail plate an endless supply of nutrients and oxygen.

The Nail Plate
This is where the magic happens. The nail plate is the part we see, admire, and polish. It may look simple, but the nail plate is more complex and multilayered than you might imagine. It is composed of over 100 layers of nail cells, keratin, and other tissues.

The Nail Side Walls
The nail side walls are the fleshy parts where the nail bed and finger skin meet. They protect the edges of the nail plate. Damage to the side walls can lead to hangnails, ingrown nails, or the flattening out of your nail bed.

NAIL GROWTH

Now that we know all the parts of the nail, the next key topic is how the nail grows. It all starts in the matrix. The top edge of the matrix is presented as the lunula. Nail plate cells are born deep in the matrix. As the cells run their course (or to put it more brutally—die), they are pushed out and change form to become flat, translucent, and hard. The oldest cells are the most compressed, so our nail plate grows harder and thicker toward the free edge. The plate grows forward on the nail bed and lies like a vertical blind. As we grow older, the nail bed produces less oil and moisture, and grooves becomes obvious as vertical ridges in the nail plate.

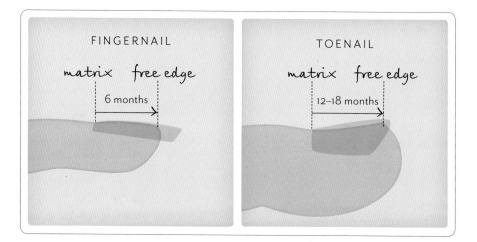

TIP: If you are trying to grow out your nails, always keep them polished. Even a simple coat of clear polish will give your nails extra support to keep breakage at bay.

Nails grow in an endless variety of shapes that vary from person to person. Some nails grow long and narrow, and others grow short and wide. Some grow slightly upward and some curve under. Some nail beds are flat and some are arched. The shape in which your nails grow is unique to you, and consistent regardless of health or diet.

A healthy adult's nails grow at a rate of approximately one-tenth of an inch per month. Nail growth slows down in winter, and speeds up in summer. Here's a strange fact: the middle fingernail grows the fastest, and the thumb grows the slowest. Freaky, right?

If you crave long, healthy nails, here is the bottom line: a healthy body leads to healthy nails. Feed your body good nutrients, and your nails will grow long and strong. Just as a car cannot run without fuel, your body can't run effectively without proper nutrition. And that hot bod of yours is smart; if deprived of fuel, it will sacrifice beauty features like glossy hair and strong nails in order to feed more important organs like your heart and brain.

So, darling, if long, strong nails are what you seek, then eat healthy foods, exercise often, and take those multivitamins!

Want whiter nails?
Eat more iron!
Leafy greens, grains,
seeds, broccoli, and
tofu are great.

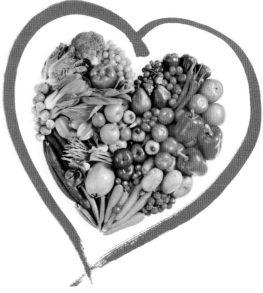

Treat your body like the temple it is! Give it only the best, inside and out.

✳ HEALTHY HANDS

Healthy, gorgeous hands are a must if you want to show off your killer nails, so be sure to give your hands plenty of TLC. We use our hands constantly, so they are the first to suffer from excess wear and tear. A bomb set of tips is useless if your hands are a wreck, so treat them well and protect them from damage.

Dryness is the primary issue that keeps hands from looking their best. If you find that your hands are always dry and chapped, try changing the soap you use. Many cleansers contain harsh sulfates that suck the moisture and life out of your skin. Try a gentle, sulfate-free cream cleanser chock-full of natural oils and moisturizers.

Washing your hands in hot water will also dry your skin, so just keep the temperature warm. While we're on the subject of water, drink plenty of it! Hydration is a must for healthy, glowing skin.

Also, remember to use sunscreen. Many of us are on point when it comes to blocking our faces from those dangerous ultraviolet rays, but too often we forget about our hands. Hands are usually the first body part to show age from sun damage. So reapply sunscreen often, especially after washing your hands. Prevention is far easier than correction.

Beautiful hands also need hand cream. Chapped, dry hands are more prone to infection because bacteria can sneak into the cracked skin more easily. The best hand creams usually come with SPF built in, so you can protect and moisturize in one easy step. Hand cream applied throughout the day will keep hands soft and flexible, so they feel as good as they look.

✳ HEALTHY FEET

Your feet are the supportive pedestals on which stands the rest of your hot bod. They take so much abuse as you pound the pavement in your trendy shoes and boots. Never wear uncomfortable footwear; doing so will only lead to corns, bunions, calluses, and just plain sore feet. Yes, foot problems can be hereditary, but bad footwear can also be a catalyst for a number of unpleasant issues.

In the winter, we tend to spend a lot of time in heavy shoes and boots. During this time, try to keep your feet dry to prevent fungus growth. You can do so by using foot powder before spending a long day in warm footwear. During the rest of the year, keeping your feet moisturized will lead to lovely heels and toes.

The best time to moisturize your feet is at night. Try covering them with a thick cream or lotion and putting on socks before bedtime. This is an amazing way to deliver a punch of moisture. Treat yourself to a pedicure at least once a week. A good soak can do wonders for tired feet. If your soles need more help than an at-home pedicure can provide, and problems persist or become painful, see a podiatrist.

HYGIENE TIPS

→ To keep your hands clean and healthy, wash them as often as you can. Think of all the public doorknobs you touch, all the hands you shake—they're all teeming with bacteria and germs. When you're on the go or between washes, make hand sanitizer your best friend and use it often.

→ For a deeper clean at home, incorporate a nail brush into your washing routine. If you can't find one in your local beauty store, a toothbrush will do. Load the brush with cleanser and scrub those pointers clean, both over and under the nail plate.

→ When you're out and about, you can carry a metal file and use that to gently scrape debris out from under your free edge. Be gentle with your skin and never use force.

→ Protect your hands from dirt whenever possible. When cleaning, dusting, gardening, or doing anything that involves getting down and dirty, wear protective gloves.

→ Shorter nails are easier to keep clean than long nails. Keeping your nails short will also help prevent you from scratching yourself (or someone else).

→ Always clean and sanitize your tools after every use.

AVOIDING INFECTION

In order to prevent infection, it is important to understand how it happens. Bacteria, fungi, and viruses sneak into the body through the mouth, nose, eyes, ears, and cut, scratched, or broken skin. Some common delivery vehicles for these bacteria, fungi, and viruses include contaminated fingers, unclean manicure water, dirty tools, and dirt, dust, and other particles inhaled through the nose and mouth.

Any nail with swelling, redness, pain, or pus could be infected. Only a doctor can treat a nail disease; if these problems persist, seek medical treatment. It is important that you never work on infected skin. Even filing can release infectious spores that may be inhaled and cause a lung infection. Bacteria can live and breed in nails tools, so you must wash, disinfect, and dry your tools after every use. Make health your top priority before styling those glamorous nails.

✳ NAIL ISSUES

The health of your nails offers clues to the health of your entire body. Healthy fingernails are firm but flexible, pinkish, and shiny. The color will vary depending on your skin tone. The surface of the nail should be smooth and free of spots, splits, or dips.

Many unsightly and uncomfortable nail conditions are minor problems, like a hangnail or a dark bruise from slamming a finger in a door. But some other nail issues indicate a deeper concern and should tell you to look at what's going on in your body. Only a doctor can diagnose medical conditions, but the chart below describes some common nail problems and potential underlying causes. When in doubt, ask your doctor.

ISSUE	CAUSE
Peeling nails	Vitamin A deficiency or dehydration
Poor nail growth	Zinc or Omega-3 deficiency
Thin, brittle nails	Poor diet
Ridges	Uneven nail growth
Dark nails	Extra melanin (skin color pigment) in the nail bed
White spots	Damage to the nail root
Bitten nails	Self-inflected damage
Frequent hangnails	Dry skin or overcutting the living tissue area
Splitting, brittle nails	Exposure to harsh chemicals
Nail plate separation from the nail bed	Trauma or allergic reaction
Ingrown nails	Improper trimming of the nail by filing or cutting the nail too deep in the corners
Green spots	Bacteria

nail trends throughout the ages

→ Ancient Times

It is said that the birth of nail art took place in India during the Bronze Age. The chic women of that era stained their nails with henna and kohl to achieve a look to make the locals stare.

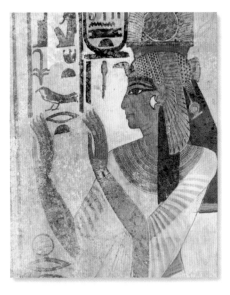

But leave it to the Egyptians to come up with the queen of all nail trends, red nails. In Queen Nefertiti's day, nail color was a symbol of status, and only royals were allowed to rock red. Cleopatra was said to sport a rusty-red color when she ruled. Even to this day, red nails signify a woman in charge!

Ancient Chinese women also loved to sass up their looks. They crushed flower petals on their nails to create new and unique colors. But just like in Egypt, there were rules stating who could wear which hue. In 600 B.C. only nobles could wear gold or silver nails, and peasants had to keep theirs pale. If a peasant dared to walk on the metallic side, the punishment would be death for impersonating a person of a higher class.

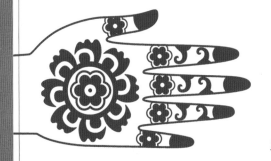

20

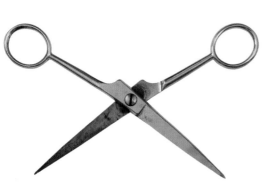

→ 1920s

It wasn't until the 1920s that the nail world received a major upgrade. During a photo shoot for a car advertisement, someone had the bright idea to take the same paint used on the car and put it on the model's nails. At that moment, the beauty world was changed forever.

→ 1930s

This was the decade of the moon manicure in all tones of red. Women believed that leaving the lunula exposed would prevent the nails from suffocating. Also in this era, Charles Revson launched the cosmetic company Revlon, which offered a new kind of nail polish based on pigments instead of dyes. The use of pigments opened up a wider range of options, creating an assortment of colors available for women to choose from. Revlon also pushed the envelope with beauty trends, making it cool to match lip color to nail color.

→ 1800s

When the 1800s brought about the technological boom known as the Industrial Revolution, new grooming tools came on the scene as well. A foot doctor in Europe invented the wooden pusher, or orangewood stick. Before the invention of this handy little stick, acid, scissors, and metal rods were used for manicures and pedicures, which only doctors performed.

Now that women were safely armed with tools to groom their nails outside of medical offices, salons began to offer nail care services. But women still usually took care of their nails by themselves. During this time, almond-shaped or slightly pointed nails were all the rage!

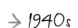

→ 1950s

In the 1950s, nails began to take a back seat to eyes. Women traded in their deep, rich, dark shades of polish for lighter, paler shades. Oval nails were still the norm, but now the hairline tip was prominent. This look was achieved by running a thumb across the tip of a freshly polished, still-wet nail.

The '50s also birthed the Juliette nail wrap manicure, named for its creator, Juliette Marglen. No longer did women need to cut up tea bags or use their husbands' cigarette papers to mend their splitting, cracked, or breaking nails. These all-natural wraps came in kits with sheets and adhesive liquid to repair or strengthen nails.

→ 1940s

In the 1940s, people began taking fashion cues from celebrities, a trend that continues today. The ever-popular red hue was still en vogue, but Rita Hayworth put a new spin on the red nail by sporting a longer, less-pointed nail. She also left the moon manicure behind and lacquered the whole nail. Legions of women followed suit. Women also began using tea bags or cigarette papers applied with glue to strengthen weak nails, or to repair broken ones.

→ 1960s

By the 1960s, red nails were completely out of style and considered old-fashioned. Delicate shades like vanilla, baby pink, and cream were the colors of choice. At this time, chicks kept their tips simple, subdued, and practical.

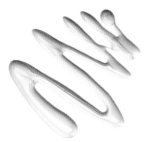

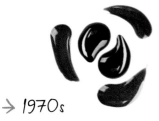

→ 1970s

The 1970s led to new nail styles and techniques, creating a renaissance in the world of nails. Square nails were all the rage, and this decade launched the acrylic nail as we know it. By the end of the '70s, nails were worn very long, thanks to the added strength of the acrylic.

Artificial press-on tips also came on the scene in the '70s. These full coverage tips could be worn only for special occasions, or just for one night. Any contact with water would deactivate the glue holding them to the nail plate, making wearing them a pain.

As the decade wore on, black nail polish became popular with punk rock and Goth kids, both male and female. In contrast, more conservative, preppy women were introduced to the French manicure.

→ 1980s

Because of the popularity of acrylic enhancements, women once again headed to the salon to get their tips done. In addition to fiberglass wrap enhancements, manicurists started offering unique hand-painted designs and charms as optional add-ons to the traditional manicure. As far as style trends went, there simply were no rules.

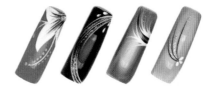

→ 1990s

With so many old and new nail grooming options available, the 1990s were a time of freedom when it came to nail style. But of course, the tried-and-true deep red nail made a major comeback. In a little film called *Pulp Fiction*, actress Uma Thurman's style made waves, and Chanel breathed new life into the classic look with its cult-classic dark red shade known as "Rouge Noir" or "Vamp."

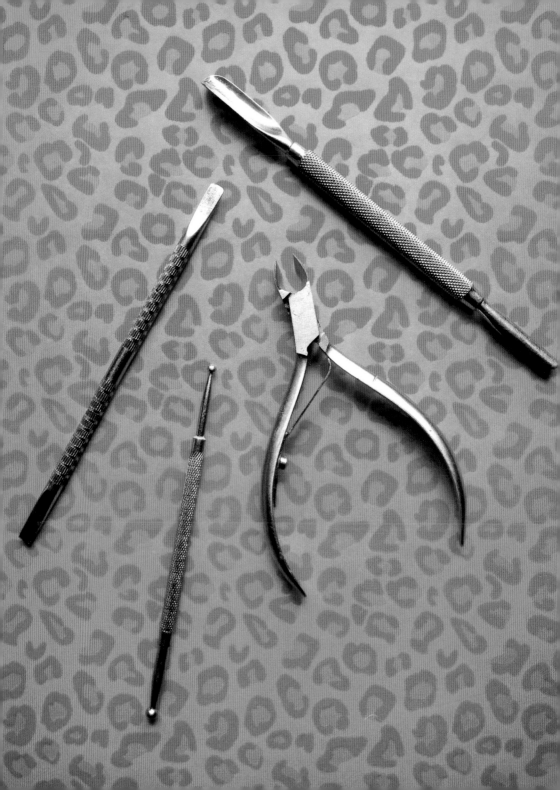

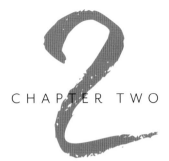

CHAPTER TWO

using the right tools

"It's not the tools that do the damage; it's the fools that do the damage."
—GREG SALO of YOUNG NAILS

The right tools are an absolute necessity,

but so is the know-how to use them correctly. If jacked-up nails are the end result of your manicure, the tools are not to blame. For a killer manicure, you need a set of basic tools and the knowledge of how to use them—the right way. Whatever tool you use, always remember to read the manufacturer's instructions and labels. A few minutes spent reading product information can save you time, stress, and even a trip to the emergency room! And always be sure to clean and sanitize your tools after every use. Now let's break down the basics and do away with self-inflicted damage. Here are all the tools you need to turn out a kick-ass manicure.

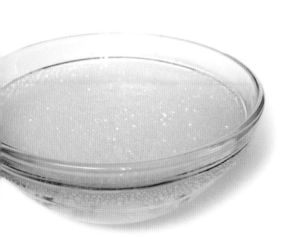

FOOT BASIN

To give your feet the royal treatment, soak them in a bath of warm, soapy water. A foot tub, or pedicure tub, is the tool for this job. These bowls are portable, flat-bottomed, and big enough to fit both feet. They are heavy when full of water; fill and empty them by hand. Allow your feet to soak for at least five minutes before smoothing and shaping. This step will clean your feet and soften your skin, making your feet easier to work on. Adding botanicals, oils, or bath salts to the water will turn a standard at-home pedicure into a luscious, spalike experience.

FINGER BOWL

Use a finger bowl to soak those gorgeous hands. Professional finger bowls are designed with grooves to rest your fingers comfortably while your nails soak. Professional bowls are also equipped with a place to rest your wrist after a long day of working. If you don't have a professional finger bowl, any bowl made of plastic, glass, or metal will work.

TOWELS

Clean towels are a must. You will use towels throughout your pampering to dry off your hands and feet after your treatment, and to wipe off products like cuticle remover, masks, and debris. Cloth towels work better, but paper towels make for easier cleanup. I also like to put a towel under the water basins (foot and hand) to catch spillage.

POLISH REMOVER

Removers break down and remove nail polish and other nail enhancements. Some removers are made of ethyl acetate and others are acetone-based. Ethyl acetate-based removers will remove only polish, and some are more effective than others. Acetone is stronger and will remove the whole shebang. One-hundred percent acetone works quickly and leaves nails completely bare and undressed. The less time your skin spends in contact with any kind of stripping agent, the better.

NAIL BRUSH

The nail brush looks like an oversized tooth brush with either a small handle or no handle at all. Used with soapy water, it fully removes dirt and germs from your fingernails. To use, just apply soap to the bristles, scrub over your nail plate and under your free edge, and then rinse the gunk away.

COTTON BALLS AND WIPES

Cotton products come in a variety of forms, including wipes and puffs. They are used mainly to remove product such as nail lacquer or enhancements. Saturate the cotton in polish remover and sweep it across the nail to remove polish. Place a soaked cotton ball or wipe on the nail plate and let it rest for a bit longer to remove gel, wraps, and acrylics.

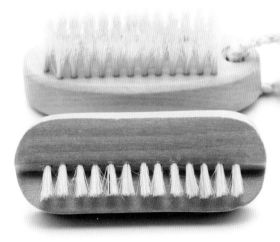

✳ NAIL FILES AND BUFFERS

Files and buffers are available in a wide range of styles. Files and buffers can be either disposable or reusable, if made of material that can be disinfected. Their grit ranges from coarse to soft. They can be flexible or rigid, large or small, and even made of glass. You can find files and buffers in a wide range of shapes and colors. Pay attention to the grit; the higher the number, the finer the grit. Finer grit means that the file or buffer is gentler and less abrasive. Low-grit boards and blocks should be handled with extreme caution and used by a professional, as they remove more tissue and product per swipe. Using a low-grit file on your own may result in excessive damage. Avoid using 80-grit files at home, and stick to 180-240–grit or higher.

To master the art of the file, first make sure the nail plate is completely dry. A wet nail plate is weak and prone to chipping and damage. Do not saw back and forth; always file in one direction. Commit this to memory! Filing back and forth, or "saw-filing," is a common mistake that causes the nail to break, chip, and snag. Saw-filing leaves the surface rough, but filing in one direction results in smoothly shaped nails.

Use a buffer after filing to smooth out the nail plate and shine it up prettily. Use caution, as excessive buffing causes damage that will build up over time. If you ever feel a burning sensation when filing or buffing, stop immediately—you're overdoing it.

Always file in one direction. Commit this to memory!

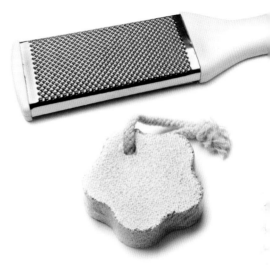

FOOT FILE

Foot files are used to smooth out the bottoms of your soles. The surface is similar to sandpaper, but like nail files, they are also available in metal and glass. My favorite foot files are two-sided. One side is coarse to remove excess hard, dry, or callused skin; the other side is soft and buffs the skin for a smooth finish.

PUMICE STONE

Like the foot file, a pumice stone is used to remove dry, dead skin, and to reduce the size of corns and calluses. Pumice stones come in a variety of colors, shapes, and sizes. After soaking your feet, dip the pumice stone in the water, and then rub it lightly on rough spots on your feet.

Keep in mind, completely smoothing out rough feet takes time and care. Be persistent; baby-soft feet will not happen on the first try. But take care and be gentle; rubbing too hard with a pumice stone or file can break the skin.

CALLUS SOFTENERS

Callus softeners are liquid gels that make smoothing out rough heels and calluses a breeze. The common active ingredients used in these treatments are lactic acid and sodium hydroxide. These two additives are very powerful because they're highly alkaline. To use, apply directly to the callus with a cotton ball or with glove-covered hands. Let it soak in for the recommended time according to the manufacturer's instructions, then thoroughly rinse off your feet and wash your hands. Now, your formerly dry, rough feet will be soft and your calluses will be easier to remove with a foot file or pumice stone.

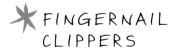

FINGERNAIL CLIPPERS

Clippers are handy when the free edges of the nail grow long and you need to take them down a notch. Clippers will save you from spending excessive time filing.

TOENAIL CLIPPERS

Toenail clippers are just a larger version of fingernail clippers. Because toenails are thicker and stronger than fingernails, you need a stronger tool to make a swift and clean cut. The larger size of the toenail clipper gives that added strength to trim toenails with ease. Toenail clippers also have a wider mouth to accommodate the thickness of the toenails.

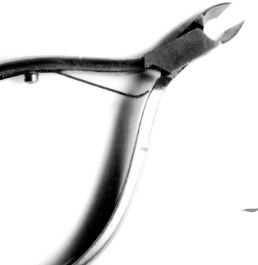

WOODEN PUSHER

The wooden pusher is used to remove excess cuticle tissue, dirt, and more from the nail. Take note: the pusher removes excess cuticle tissue, not *all* of the cuticle! Remember, cuticles are there for a reason, so you must fight any urge to abuse them. To use the wooden pusher, hold it like a pencil and gently glide it down the nail plate toward the base in a scooping motion, lifting and removing dead tissue as you go. The scooping motion should feel like shoveling snow.

NIPPERS

When using nippers, consider the famous line from *Spider-Man:* "With great power comes great responsibility." Nippers are sharp and powerful, and must be used with caution. Use nippers to trim away dead skin tags that hang off or stick up from the nail plate. Never use nippers to cut living tissue, as this will cause damage. Cuts lead to scabs that result in rough, scaly, cracked skin, which leads to more cutting. Avoid this vicious cycle!

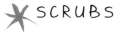

NOTE: Hair conditioner makes a great cuticle conditioner! Rub a little on your fingers, wait ten minutes, and rinse.

✳ CUTICLE REMOVER

Cuticle remover dissolves dead tissue from the nail plate, or loosens it for easier removal. Most cuticle removers are made up of 5 percent gentle acids. Be sure to use cuticle removers as directed to prevent skin damage, and to ensure that your cuticles keep working their magic to protect the rest of your skin.

✳ SCRUBS

Scrubs are used to treat dry, flaky skin and calluses by removing dead skin cells through exfoliation. Usually, coarse grains are added to lotion or body butter. These exfoliation grains come in a variety of forms, including, salt, sugar, ground seeds, and plastic beads. To use a scrub, just rub it gently on wet skin, then rinse. Be warned that overscrubbing can cause major damage to living skin, so always read the labels and use as directed.

✳ NAIL OIL AND MOISTURIZER

Moisture is essential to healthy, beautiful nails. Nail moisturizers come in cream, oil, and gel form. Their function is to hydrate and penetrate the nails and the skin around them. Moisturizers help reduce dryness in brittle nails, and increase flexibility in hard nails.

✳ HAND AND FOOT MOISTURIZER

You cannot complete a mani-pedi without the finishing touch of added moisture to your hands and feet. Creams and lotions designed for the hands and feet are denser than body moisturizers because the skin on your hands and feet is the thickest. Use moisturizer after you clean and shape your nails, but before you prep them for polish. When you prepare your nails for polish, you will want to remove the trace oils left on the nail plate by the moisturizer to ensure your polish stays put longer.

✳ NAIL TIPS

If you can't wait for your natural nails to grow long, or they won't inch up to your desired length, artificial tips are the solution. Tips come in all shapes and sizes, including square, oval, pointed, and duck-billed. They are used as a foundation for wraps, gel, and acrylic. In general, tips should not cover more than one-third of your natural nail plate. However, if you want to glam it up for one night, you can try full-coverage tips.

Tips are also designed with a variety of well shapes. The well is the curved underside of the tip that hugs your natural nail. Think of the well as a guideline or contact zone where the artificial tip meets your nail bed. The well is also the area where you apply your nail glue. You can find full-well, half-well or well-less tips. The free edge must fill the well to ensure proper placement and security of the plastic tip. Once applied, the artificial tip must be blended flush to the natural nail using a buffer. The smaller the well, the less time you will spend blending. Well-less tips are thinner and don't require any blending at all.

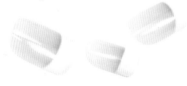

✳ NAIL GLUE

Nail glue acts as a bonder. It fixes cracks, repairs breaks, and adheres the tip to the nail. Glues come in many forms, including brush-on, squeeze tubes, liquids, and gels, and can be clear or pink in tone.

Nail glue can be used in a pinch to temporarily correct lifting of enhancements, such as acrylics, until you can make it home or to the salon for proper removal. Before using nail glue, make sure your hands and nails are dry—any moisture trapped in the nail before gluing could lead to fungus.

✳ TOE SEPARATORS

Toe separators are pieces of foam with grooves for your toes. They help create space between each toe to prevent them from smudging one another while the polish dries. Put them on before you polish to keep toenails smudge-free.

✳ SANDALS AND THONGS

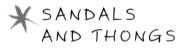

Open-toed footwear after a pedicure is key for keeping your feet clean and your polish perfect while it dries.

cleaning your tools

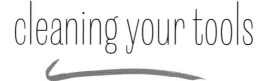

If tools aren't properly cleaned, bacteria and fungus will simply run wild. Every tool should be fully cleaned and sterilized after every use. Washing with soap and water is not enough, if you really want to remain germ-free. Follow these steps to keep your metal nippers, clippers, foot files, and other reusable implements pristine.

1) Wash tools by hand with antibacterial soap under running water. Use a nail brush or toothbrush to scrub out all dirt and product buildup from tool crevices. Make sure you don't use this brush for anything but tool cleaning.

2) Rinse and dry tools.

3) Sterilize tools using one of the following methods:

→ Preheat an oven to 375 degrees Fahrenheit. Place the tools on a foil-lined cookie sheet in the oven for 15 minutes. Remove from the oven and let sit until the tools have cooled.

→ Fully submerge the tools in a pot of boiling water for 20 minutes. Pour the contents of the pot into a strainer and let sit until the tools have cooled.

4) Place your freshly cleaned implements in an airtight bag. Never store dirty tools with clean ones.

NOTE: Most tools made of porous or absorbent material, such as files, buffers, and wooden pushers, are designed for one-time use only. Do not attempt to disinfect these items unless they are clearly labeled with information for disinfecting. If you're not sure, be safe and discard after use.

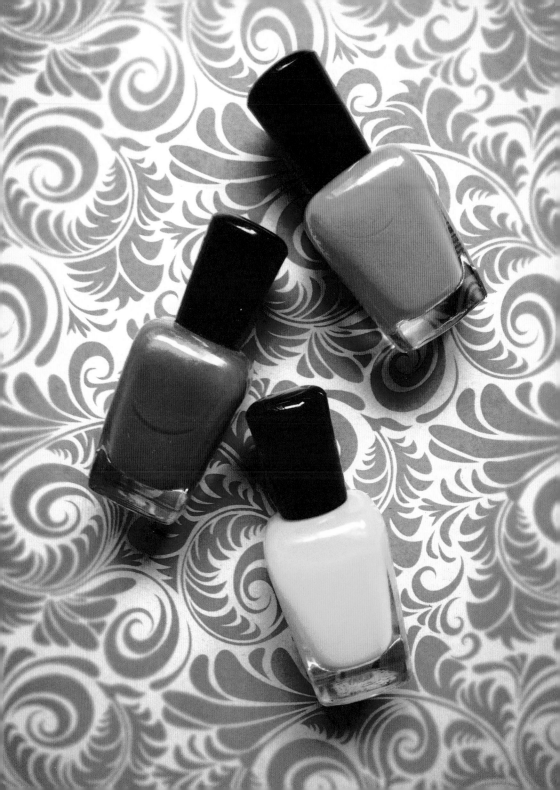

nail polish and enhancements

How do you pick your polish? With hundreds of brands, thousands of finishes, and millions of colors, you could spend all day choosing the perfect one to grace your tips. Entering a beauty store to choose a nail polish can be daunting because of the seemingly endless array of shades and formulations out there. Add to that the lure of brand labels, catchy names, and stellar marketing. How can you not want to collect them all? Talk about a dilemma. And what about a base coat and a top coat? Do all these products have different uses, and do you really need them? Well, knowledge is power, so here is the information you need to navigate the racks upon racks of polish.

✶ BASE COATS AND TREATMENTS

What does a base coat do? Most quality base coats contain nutrients to replenish damaged nails: protein, aloe vera, vitamin E, and calcium. A base coat also holds the nail polish onto the nail plate, and at the same time, prevents the polish from staining the nails. It may sometimes seem like a pain to go that extra step, but applying a base coat will extend the life of your manicure. Whether you're going for a vampy red or rock-Goth black, base coat will keep your nails from being stained. So bite the bullet; it only takes two minutes to apply, tops! Now, let's break down the different types of base coats.

Classic Base Coat

Classic base coat is the key to a long-lasting manicure. It is colorless and does the basic job of anchoring your color polish to the nail plate and keeping your natural nails stain-free.

MY TOP THREE BASE COATS

Based on drying time and chip resistance

1) Zoya Anchor Base Coat

2) Butter London Nail Foundation

3) CND Stickey Base Coat

Nail Hardener/Strengthener

Nail hardener is a coating placed directly on the natural nail. A hardening or strengthening base coat adds some extra oomph to help your nails become stronger and harder. Most of the time, that extra help comes from formaldehyde. But, no need to worry about toxicity; formaldehyde molecules are too big to creep through the nail plate and into your body. The strong bond created by formaldehyde helps weak nails become stiffer and less prone to breakage. But please be warned: if after adding this product to your nail-care routine, you see your nails starting to change color or become dry and flaky, stop using it immediately. This type of hardener is not for everyone. Instead, try a formaldehyde-free formula that uses calcium, protein, silk, or gel.

MY TOP THREE HARDENERS/STRENGTHENERS

1) Nail Tek Intensive Therapy II

2) Develop 10 Ultimate Nail Strengthening Formula

3) Kur Nail Hardener

Nail Hydrator

Nail hydrators are made for dry, brittle, inflexible nails. They are filled with oils, soy, aloe, or other kinds of moisture to help bring life back to dehydrated nails.

MY TOP THREE HYDRATORS

1) Deborah Lippmann Hard Rock Hydrating Nail Hardener

2) Ciaté Nail Tonic Hydrator

3) Sephora by OPI Hydrator

Ridge Filler

Ridge filler does just what it says. It fills the ridges and wrinkles on the nail plate, giving the nail a smoother appearance. Ridge filler tends to be thicker than other types of nail treatments because it needs the extra body to mask the uneven imperfections in the nail. Ingredients vary from one brand to another. Use trial and error to find out which one works for you.

MY TOP THREE RIDGE FILLERS

1) Essie Fill The Gap! Ridge Smoothing Base Coat

2) Nail Tek Foundation Ridge Filling Nail Strengthener

3) Zoya Get Even Ridge Filling Base Coat

Growth Treatment

Nail growth treatments are little potions designed to support quicker natural nail growth, made with active ingredients proven to nourish the nail and nail bed. Some common ingredients are biotin, omega-3 acids, green tea, calcium, keratin, peptides, and a slew of others. Each growth treatment is unique due to the variety of ingredients used.

MY TOP THREE GROWTH TREATMENTS

1) Sally Hansen Nailgrowth Miracle Serum

2) GoNails Natural Nail Growth Treatment

3) Mavala Mavaderma Nail Growth Treatment

Cosmetic brands are churning out new treatments every day in a never-ending quest for the perfect formula to solve all nail problems. So get out there and start swiping until you get the results you desire.

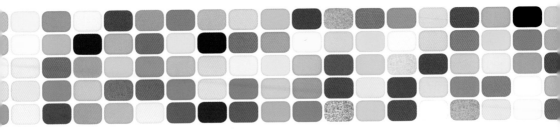

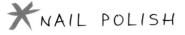NAIL POLISH

You can call it lacquer, varnish, enamel, or polish, but the last thing you can call it is boring. Polish is the main ingredient that delivers your desired look. Polish is used for a number of things:

→ to cover imperfections or discoloring

→ to strengthen the nails

→ to protect the nails

→ to complement a makeup look or outfit

→ just because you love it!

Polish ingredients are generally the same, regardless of the brand: nitrocellulose, or film former; resins to add hardness and shine; and pigment for color. Glitter or iridescence is often included for extra flash. All these ingredients are living in a little glass bottle, just waiting to be applied to the nail with a brush. The purpose is to bring a temporary visual POW! to your fingers and toes.

MY TOP THREE POLISH BRANDS

Based on color payoff, lasting power, drying time, and originality

1) Zoya

2) Deborah Lippman

3) Butter London

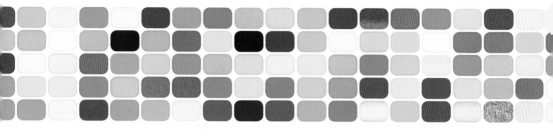

★ TOP COAT

Once color is applied to your liking, it's time to top it all off. Top coat is the cherry on top of all this glamour. Made primarily of acrylic, top coat dries to a hard finish, creating a chip-, peel-, and scratch-resistant surface. Reapplying top coat every other day will leave you with a manicure that goes the distance.

When selecting a top coat, consider what kind of finish you are looking for. The most sought-after top coats dry quickly. These "quick-dry" lacquers are made with the same ingredients as the pigmented polishes, but with a different ratio. Their goal is to leave your nails shiny and smudge-proof in a small amount of time.

MY TOP THREE TOP COATS

Based on drying time, glossiness, and chip-resistance

1) Deborah Lippmann Addicted to Speed Ultra Quick-Dry Top Coat

2) Seche Vite Dry Fast Top Coat

3) Sally Hansen Insta-Dri Anti-Chip Top Coat

Now that nail art is booming, you can find many different styles of top coat. Newer top coats can come in matte finish, or with added glitter or iridescent qualities. These add-ons—like mica, crushed pearls, or titanium dioxide—give your polish color a whole new dimension while still letting your base color shine through.

QUICK-DRY TREAMENTS

Short on time, or just low on patience? Don't let that stop you from attending to your tips.

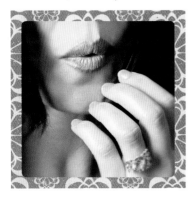

Let's get real: remember to use the powder room before you polish! (Even if you don't need to.) There is nothing worse than ruining your perfect polish while you struggle to button your jeans.

A quick-dry treatment is an optional final step that speeds up the drying time of your lacquer layers. The most accessible forms come in sprays and (my favorite) drops. These products are usually marketed with numerous claims: they instantly dry your polish; you'll be out the door in no time; polish dries completely in 60 seconds . . . blah, blah, blah! To my knowledge there has never been a quick-dry polish, drop, or spray that totally eliminates drying time. Do they reduce drying time? Yes. But get rid of it altogether? No way. Quick-dry treatments just add a protective layer of alcohol-laced silicones to lessen your chances of smudging while helping your polish evaporate. We would all love to cut down on drying time, and some quick-dry products work extremely well while others fall flat. But the truth is, there is no way you're getting away smudge-free in less than a minute.

MY TOP THREE QUICK-DRY TREATMENTS

1) Zoya Fast Drops Drying Drops

2) CND SolarSpeed Spray

3) China Glaze Fast Freeze Quick Dry Spray

Chipping Polish?
Here's Why:

→ applying polish too thinly

→ using your nails as tools

→ overusing quick-dry products

→ skipping base coat

→ dehydrated nail beds

Peeling Polish?
Here's Why:

→ not prepping the nail plate to remove surface oils

→ applying polish too thickly

→ oversoaking nails and not letting them dry fully before application

→ not allowing enough drying time between coats of color

→ skipping top coat

✳ POLISH, WRAPS, AND GEL

Here is a quick rundown of the most popular nail décor options, and some pros and cons to help you choose.

Traditional Polish

By now, you know and love your nail polish. And luckily, we live in an era where we have access to more colors and textures than ever before. I don't know a single girl who doesn't own at least one bottle of polish, even if its only clear.

PROS	CONS
→ Touch up chips on the go	→ Long drying time (It takes about 12 hours for polish to FULLY dry!)
→ Easy to find (Every pharmacy, discount store, beauty supplier, and most supermarkets carry some brand of polish.)	→ Smudging
	→ Fumes
	→ Too many chemicals
→ An inexpensive way to wear designer labels	→ It's difficult to paint your dominant hand
→ Unlimited colors available, with more coming out each day	→ It's difficult to keep polish from getting on your cuticles
→ Easy to maneuver, which makes it great for nail art	

Nail Wraps

Nail wraps are flexible pieces of polymer or acrylic film that are applied to the nails like stickers. (Remember, polish is also a form of acrylic.) Some brands require a heating device to set them to your nail, while others let you stick and go! Every female celeb I know loves to rock nail wraps. Beyoncé, Katy Perry, Pink, Lady Gaga, and Rihanna have all been seen on the scene sporting this easy option.

PROS	CONS
→ No smudging	→ Your natural body chemistry affects their staying power
→ No drying time	
→ More complex looks than you can achieve with polish, such as metallic or chrome	→ They don't last long on artificial tips
	→ They can get expensive! A bottle of polish can last you a very long time, but wraps are for one-time use only.
→ No fumes	
→ No bleeding onto your cuticles	→ Pre-cut wraps won't always fit every nail shape
→ Your dominant and nondominant hands come out looking equally good	

Gel polish

Gel polish is a hybrid of traditional nail polish and soak-off gel enhancements. It brushes on like polish, and each layer must be cured or hardened under a UV or LCD light, depending on the brand.

PROS	CONS
→ If properly applied, you will have a chip-free manicure for at least two weeks	→ Longer application time
	→ For the best results, you must buy the whole system
→ Most brands have been proven to promote healthy nail growth	
	→ If improperly applied, this polish won't last
→ No need to be on smudge alert; after your application is complete, you are good to go!	
	→ If improperly applied, you risk damage to the nail plate
→ More natural-looking than gel tips	
→ Lightweight	

✳ CHOOSING COLORS

This story has happened to all of us: you hunt through the nail polish rack until you come across the most beautiful color, ever. Everything about it, from the color to the finish, is puuurrrr-fect. So you buy it, take it home for a test drive and . . . it looks terrible when you put it on. Why is that?

Well, simply put, the color did not play well with your skin tone. Your skin tone is fabulous and perfect exactly the way it is. But when you make a meal, you must choose side dishes to complement the main dish, not compete with it. There is a reason why you'll never see McDonald's serving burgers with a side of nachos. We all know how delicious both can be, but together, they do not work! Use the same philosophy when choosing colors to complement your skin tone. Beauty comes in all colors, and so does nail enamel. The key is finding the hues that work for you. Follow these tips, and you'll see you can't judge a polish by the bottle.

Consider Your Undertone

Look carefully at your skin. Does it have a cool or warm tint to it that radiates from within? Undertones fall into two main categories: pink and yellow. When picking jewelry, which metals do you gravitate toward? If your answer is silver or white gold, your undertone is most likely pink. If your answer is yellow gold, you're probably a girl with a yellow undertone. Team Pink ladies will look best in blue-based colors and Team Yellow ladies look best in coral or orange-based colors.

Consider the Season

Nail colors, like fashion styles, are seasonal. In the winter, our complexions tend to get paler and richer, and darker color seems to suit us more. Once the heat of summer kicks in, turn to a brighter, flirtier color.

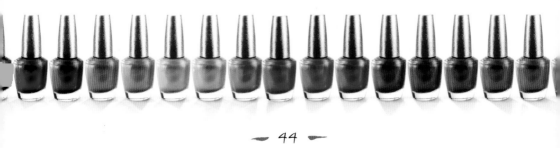

MUST-TRY COLORS FOR EVERY SKIN TONE

- MAC Nail Lacquer in Mean & Green
- Butter London in Yummy Mummy
- Ginger + Liz in Swagger
- Deborah Lippmann in Happy Birthday
- Deborah Lippmann in Sugar Daddy
- Zoya in Wednesday
- Essie in Bermuda Shorts

NOTE: You know dark colors make your waistline look smaller, but did you know they make your nails look smaller too? Choose light colors to create the illusion of length, or use my favorite lengthening trick: leave a tiny border around your cuticle and along the sides of the nail. This optical illusion creates a frame for the nail, making it look longer.

porcelain skin

SHADES TO CHOOSE

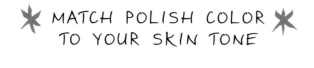

Reds that fall in the wine and oxblood family.
Nudes that are mauve or soft-blush in tone.
Pinks that are silver, rosy, or ashy.

SHADES TO AVOID

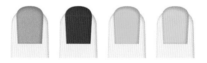

Orange, brown, yellow, and peach.

MY TOP 5 CONSERVATIVE COLORS FOR PORCELAIN SKIN
Use these shades when you need to be professional at work or school.

	MAC Nail Lacquer in Angel
	Sally Hansen Complete Salon Manicure in Shell We Dance
	Yves Saint Laurent La Laque Couture in Rose Romantique
	Essie in Mademoiselle
	Essie in Sugar Daddy

MY TOP 5 OUTRAGEOUS COLORS FOR PORCELAIN SKIN
Use these shades when you want to make people do a double-take.

	Essie in Stylenomics
	Orly in Skinny Dip
	MAC Nail Lacquer in Girl Trouble
	Essie in Chinchilly
	Nars in Schiap

MY TOP 5 REDS FOR PORCELAIN SKIN
Use these shades to make the ultimate feminine statement.

	Nars in Jungle Red
	OPI in Big Apple Red
	OPI in I'm Not Really a Waitress
	Dior Diorific Vernis in Marilyn
	MAC Nail Lacquer in Shirelle

olive skin

SHADES TO CHOOSE

Reds that fall in the rusty-warm family.
Nudes that are caramel-brown or peach.
Pinks that are yellow-based or golden in tone.

SHADES TO AVOID

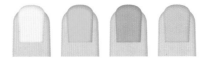

Soft pinks and blue-grays.

MY TOP 5 CONSERVATIVE COLORS FOR OLIVE SKIN
Use these shades when you need to be professional at work or school.

	Zoya in Lulu
	MAC Nail Lacquer in Skin
	Chanel in Frenzy
	Essie in Not Just a Pretty Face
	Essie in Sugar Daddy

MY TOP 5 OUTRAGEOUS COLORS FOR OLIVE SKIN
Use these shades when you want to make people do a double-take.

	Chanel in June
	MAC Nail Lacquer in Girl About Town
	Yves Saint Laurent La Laque Couture in Khaki Arty
	Obsessive Compulsive Cosmetics Nail Lacquer in Anime
	Zoya in Charisma

MY TOP 5 REDS FOR OLIVE SKIN
Use these shades to make the ultimate feminine statement.

	Revlon Top Speed in Fire
	Nars in Chinatown
	MAC Nail Lacquer in Kid Orange
	Essie in Geranium
	Essie in Russian Roulette

ebony skin

SHADES TO CHOOSE

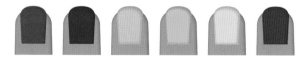

Reds, including raspberry, plum, and burgundy.
Nudes that are orange or bronze in tone.
Pinks that are caramel or rich brown.

SHADES TO AVOID

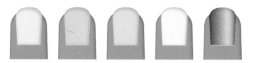

Pale colors, ashy colors, and silver.

MY TOP 5 CONSERVATIVE COLORS FOR EBONY SKIN
Use these shades when you need to be professional at work or school.

	OPI in Toasted Almond
	Chanel Le Vernis in Beige
	Deborah Lippmann in Modern Love
	Lime Crime in Milky Way
	Essie in Fiji

MY TOP 5 OUTRAGEOUS COLORS FOR EBONY SKIN
Use these shades when you want to make people do a double-take.

	Yves Saint Laurent La Laque Couture in Bleu Majorelle
	Sally Hansen Insta-Dry in Lightening
	Chanel Le Vernis in Diwali
	Essie in Fruit Sangria
	Lime Crime in Lavendairy

MY TOP 5 REDS FOR EBONY SKIN
Use these shades to make the ultimate feminine statement.

	Dolce & Gabbana Intense Nail Lacquer in Shocking
	OPI in Tasmanian Devil Made Me Do It
	Essie in Really Red
	Zoya in America
	Obsessive Compulsive Cosmetics Nail Lacquer in Vintage

✳ CRAFT STORE FINDS

I never met a craft store I didn't like; they're like a mothership for artistic souls. Yes, they sell paints, scrapbooking tools, yarn, and jewelry-making supplies, but they are more than your Nana's favorite place to shop. Surprisingly, craft stores are the best places to discover fresh new ideas and options for nail art!

To choose the best nail art supplies, you must scan the craft store aisles with the eye of a nail artist. Open your mind; look for items that are small enough to fit on your fingertips, or can be cut down to size. Check for items that can leave imprints, create cool textures, or make a good stencil. Following are some nail art ideas for you to try, using treasures from your local crafting boutique. These ideas are just a starting point; use your creativity to explore options and create unique designs!

Crystals

When choosing bling for your nails, consider the end result you're looking for. Not all crystals are created equal. Look for flat-back crystals that can be easily attached to the nail plate.

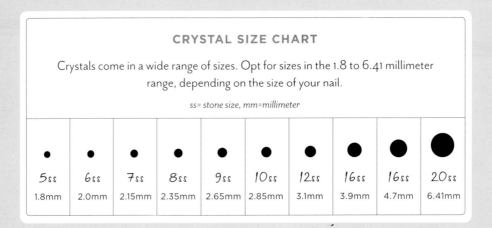

CRYSTAL SIZE CHART

Crystals come in a wide range of sizes. Opt for sizes in the 1.8 to 6.41 millimeter range, depending on the size of your nail.

ss= stone size, mm=millimeter

5ss	6ss	7ss	8ss	9ss	10ss	12ss	16ss	16ss	20ss
1.8mm	2.0mm	2.15mm	2.35mm	2.65mm	2.85mm	3.1mm	3.9mm	4.7mm	6.41mm

CRYSTAL COLOR CHART

There are no rules when it comes to color. It all depends on the look you're going for. Below are some options to choose from.

crystal	moonlight	silver shade	black diamond	jet	comet argent	alabaster
white opal	crystal ab	silk	greige	golden shadow	lt. colorado topaz	copper
topaz	smoky topaz	mocha	light peach	jonquil	light topaz	citrine
sunflower	sun	hyacinth	light siam	red magma	siam	vintage rose
rose water opal	light rose	rose	indian pink	fuschia	padparad-scha	ruby
burgundy	light amethyst	amethyst	provence lavender	violet	tanzanite	purple velvet
heliotrope	cobalt	bermuda	air blue opal	light sapphire	sapphire	capri
dark indigo	indicolite	blue zircon	caribbean blue opal	aqua	light azore	pacific opal
chrysolite opal	chrysolite	erinite	peridot	olivine	fern green	emerald

When choosing a shape, think beyond the circle. Crystals come in a wide range of shapes with which you can experiment.

MY FAVORITE CRYSTAL SHAPES				
circle	square	teardrop	heart	crescent
star	butterfly	rectangle	oval	navette

So, what makes a great crystal? Look beyond the words on the package. A good crystal sparkles to perfection every time the light hits it, even dim light. There are three types of crystals available on the market, and knowing the difference among these will make a major difference in the finished look of your nail art.

PLASTIC

These are the easiest to come by. You'll find them in beauty supply stores, drug stores, and discount stores. They are often dull, sloppily cut, and overpriced. They are best for practice or for use on kids.

GLASS

Glass rhinestones will sparkle more than a plastic rhinestone could dream of. They are a cool and affordable nail art option, so you can experiment without breaking the bank.

REAL CRYSTAL

Nothing, and I mean nothing, beats the gleam of real crystal rhinestones. Swarovski crystals are the industry standard and my favorite, mainly because of their patented multi-faceted cut. The way they catch the light is unparalleled; they really deliver the bling!

Rhinestones and crystals are best applied with tweezers on top of complete nail polish and painted nail art. Here are a few methods to adhere the stones to your nail.

Top Coat
Apply clear top coat. Using tweezers, place the stone onto the wet surface, flat side down. Gently press the stone into place. This method is super-easy, but don't plan for the stones to stay on for very long.

Adhesive
Using tweezers, pick up crystal and apply nail art glue to the flat back. Place it on the desired location on a dry nail. Be careful, because once you place it, it cannot be moved. With care, this method will last for a week or more.

Top Coat and Adhesive
Combine the two methods and apply the gem with nail glue while the top coat is still wet.

Gel
Another popular method involves embedding the stone into a gel top coat and curing it under UV or LCD light. This method has the most staying power; once set in gel, the gems won't come off until you take them off.

Some nail artists choose to paint a coat of clear top coat or gel over the gems for more staying power, but I strongly advise against this. Even a clear coat will alter the stone's facets and prevent the light from creating that desired sparkle and bling.

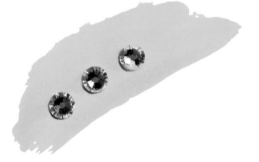

Studs

Studs with flat backs can be applied just like crystals, but they create a totally different effect; nothing says badass like studs! If you're looking for a metallic, edgy kick to your look, studs are a great nail art add-on. They also come in many sizes, styles, and finishes in addition to the standard gold and silver.

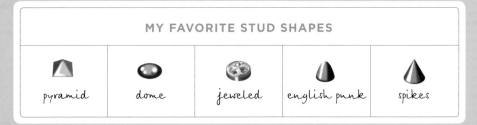

MY FAVORITE STUD SHAPES

| pyramid | dome | jeweled | english punk | spikes |

Pearls

If you're more of a soft and sweet, pretty-in-pink kind of babe, pearls are a perfect fit for you. Yes, pearls are classy and elegant, but they can also be trendy. Pearls create a luminescent effect without being over-the-top flashy. There are three types of pearls commonly in use today: natural pearls, which are found in wild oysters; cultured pearls, which are grown by farm-raised oysters; and plastic pearl replicas.

For nail art, plastic pearls are the best option because they are cheaper and easier to find. They are also much lighter in weight, so they are less likely to fall off. Unlike plastic rhinestones, plastic pearls have a similar finish and luster as real pearls. When it comes to color and shape, the list of options is nearly endless. Below are some of my favorites!

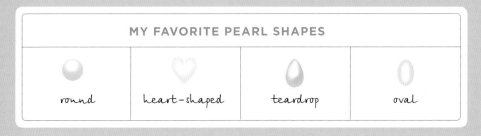

MY FAVORITE PEARL SHAPES

| round | heart-shaped | teardrop | oval |

Studs and pearls are applied in the same manner as crystals, using top coat, adhesive, or gel. Be sure to choose ones with flat backs. Try combining studs, pearls, and crystals for a unique look!

PEARL COLOR OPTIONS

white	cream	creamrose light	creamrose
gold	bright gold	copper	coral
brown	deep brown	bronze	peach
powder almond	rosaline	powder rose	mauve
burgundy	bordeaux	maroon	dark purple
night blue	light blue	tahitian look	powder green
light green	antique brass	dark green	platinum
light gray	dark gray	black	mystic black

Fabric and Lace

Fabric and lace can really take your nail art to another level! Incorporating these elements will definitely leave you with "notice-me" nails. With the guidelines in this book and some practice, you will be able to re-create the pattern of any lace or fabric you desire, but why not try the real thing? As an added bonus, unlike nail polish, fabric won't chip. Before you begin any method of application, you'll need to cut your fabric. The most accurate way to do this is to make a stencil. To make a stencil, take a piece of tissue paper and wrap it around your finger. Using a pencil, trace around your nail plate, letting your cuticle act as a guide. Repeat with each nail, then cut the stencils out, keeping track of the order. Use the stencils to cut the fabric to the right shape and size for each nail. Keep track of the order so you can match the right piece of fabric to nail. Now you'll choose a method to adhere fabric to nail.

Top Coat

Apply base coat and optional color polish, then let dry. Apply your thickest top coat. (I like Seche Vite.) While the top coat is still tacky, apply the fabric or lace with tweezers and align. Reapply top coat using the brush to gently push the fabric or lace into the nail plate. Let it dry, trim off any loose strings, then apply one or two more layers of top coat until the fabric is saturated and glossy. This method works particularly well with lace.

Mod Podge

Make sure your nail plate is clean and dry. I also like to wipe the nails clean with a mild acetone or nail dehydrator for extra lasting power. Using a small paintbrush, apply a thin layer of Mod Podge to the nail plate and let it dry just until it is a little tacky. Apply the fabric with tweezers and align, gently pressing the fabric into the glue. Apply another layer of Mod Podge, let it dry, and trim off any loose strings. Apply top coat.

There's no need to stop here—get creative and play with different shapes, cutouts, and locations of fabric!

Glitter

Glitter polish has been a cult favorite for years, because it's so beautiful that it's almost magical! When I see glitter, I just can't take my eyes off the sparkly speckles. Nails are the perfect canvas for glitter; with every flick of the hand, glitter-enhanced nails catch the light and sparkle. For a demure look, apply just a touch of glitter over neutral-colored nails. For a flashy look, go big and intense with color and size! Check out the variety of glitter sizes and colors in this handy chart.

GLITTER SIZE CHART

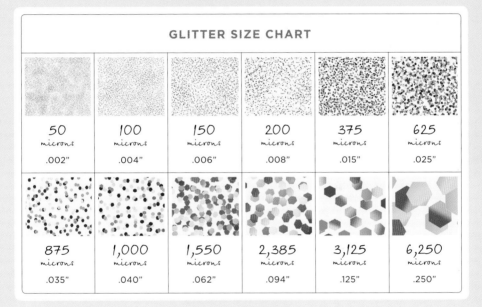

50 microns .002"	100 microns .004"	150 microns .006"	200 microns .008"	375 microns .015"	625 microns .025"
875 microns .035"	1,000 microns .040"	1,550 microns .062"	2,385 microns .094"	3,125 microns .125"	6,250 microns .250"

GLITTER FUN SHAPES

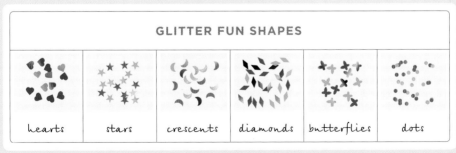

hearts	stars	crescents	diamonds	butterflies	dots

Three ways to get that pop and sparkle from glitter

THE SHAKE METHOD

Apply base coat and your desired polish color and let dry. Open the container of loose glitter and place a paper towel over your work area. Apply top coat to your nails. Shake the glitter onto wet nails over a paper towel. Use a dry, stiff paintbrush to flick away the excess glitter from the skin around your nails. Apply another layer of top coat. Be sure to wipe off the brush after each swipe to prevent the bottle from getting contaminated by wayward glitter pieces. (You may want to reserve a separate bottle of top coat just for use with glitter!)

THE DIP METHOD

Apply base coat and your desired polish color and let dry. Pour some loose glitter into a dish. Apply top coat and dip nails into the glitter, one at a time. Use your wooden pusher or orangewood stick to scoop the glitter on to the nail to make sure the plate is completely covered. Use a dry, stiff paint brush to flick away the excess glitter from the skin around your nails. Apply another layer of top coat. Again, be sure to wipe off the brush after each swipe to prevent the bottle from getting contaminated by way-ward glitter pieces.

CINDERELLA GLITTER POLISH

I like to call this the Cinderella manicure because it only lasts for one night. This method is for the girl who wants to rock glitter for a special event, but hates taking it off. All you need is Elmer's school glue! Before applying, lightly buff your nails to remove the shine. Squeeze a bit of glue onto a paper towel. Using a clean, dry nail art brush, apply the glue to your nails as you would a base coat. Flat brushes work best here. Once the glue is dry, apply glitter polish. Apply top coat and let dry. Your sparkly manicure will look perfect for at least 24 hours! To remove, use a cuticle pusher to gently pry the glitter off the nail plate. The glitter polish should come off in one full piece! No excessive soaking or rubbing needed.

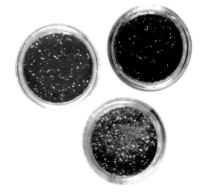

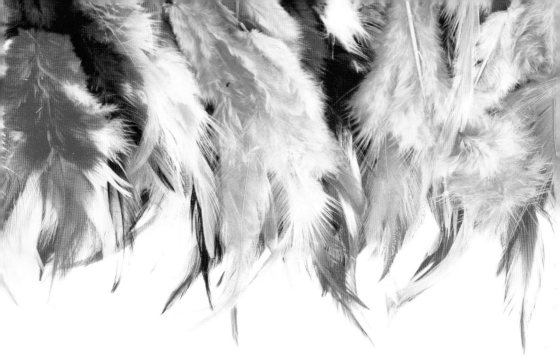

Feathers

If you want to create a more bohemian style, like celebrities Nicole Richie and Sienna Miller, put aside the glitz and glam it up with feathers in your nail art! You can find bags of feathers at any craft store. Give yourself plenty of options and buy a bag of assorted feathers. Most variety bags contain a mix of peacock, hen, cockatiel, parakeet, turkey, goose, and other feathers. No two feathers are exactly alike; choose ones that highlight your personal style. Natural, undyed feathers are very boho-chic, and dyed feathers are fun if you crave a pop of color. Feathers give a natural, organic feel to your look, and that link to nature is what makes them so enchanting. This design is decorative, yet still clean and sharp, and you'll never look the same twice!

To apply, select your feathers and apply base coat. Apply top coat to one nail, carefully glide the tip of a feather onto it, and gently press to adhere. Repeat with each nail until all are complete and let dry. Trim off the excess with cuticle scissors. Apply another layer of top coat, using a tap and glide motion, and let dry. You may want to apply one or two more layers of top coat to really seal in the feather and smooth out the look.

Tape

Let's talk tape. This wonderful invention has endless uses for a nail artist! You can find tape just about anywhere, and it's amazing for picking up spilled or out-of-control glitter on tables, clothes, and floors. You can create nail art using anything from duct tape to electrical tape, but here I'll show you how to turn out some striking designs using everyday office tape.

NEGATIVE SPACE NAIL ART

Apply base coat and let dry. Tear off a two-inch piece of tape and cut it lengthwise into six or more thin strips. Lay a few strips on your nail plate, creating a cool pattern with plenty of open space. Don't completely cover the nail with tape. Once you have an interesting design, firmly press the tape down. Paint two coats of polish color on one nail and gently peel the tape off while the polish is still wet. Repeat with each nail. Let dry completely and apply top coat.

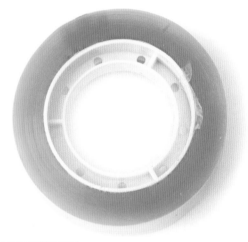

CUSTOM STICKERS

Apply base coat and two coats of color polish. Let dry. Take an array of polish colors and paint them on a few strips of tape. Let them dry. Cut the tape in tiny shapes small enough to fit onto your nail plate. Using tweezers, apply the stickers to your nail and firmly press them into place. Apply top coat and let dry.

STENCILS

Apply base coat and two coats of color polish. Let dry completely. Tear off a piece of tape and cut into the shape of your choice. Position the tape on your nail as desired and gently press into place. Working on one nail at a time, paint the portion of nail that is not covered with tape, using a different polish color from the base color. Then immediately remove the tape. Repeat with each nail. Let dry and apply top coat.

Paper

Walk down any stationery aisle and you'll find some of the most beautiful details and intricate illustrations available. Paper is great for nail art because it is inexpensive and incredibly easy to find. You may even have a few scraps tucked in a drawer somewhere because they are too pretty to throw away. Craft stores tend to have the best selection, but you can find beautiful pieces of paper everywhere! There's no sense keeping these stunning sheets tucked away in a drawer. Use one of the tutorials below to display them on your nails. No steady hands needed.

TISSUE PAPER AND WRAPPING PAPER

Choose a beautiful piece of tissue paper or wrapping paper and cut it to the shape of your nails. Try your best to keep them in order. Apply base coat and one coat of color polish. (For an extra pop, try a metallic color!) While the polish is still tacky, press the paper onto the nail plate, then let the polish dry completely. Once dry, use a high-grit (180+) or glass nail file and softly file the excess paper off the free edge of the nail. Gently apply top coat in a "tap-and-glide" motion, then let dry.

LASER-PRINTED PAPER TRANSFER

Using a laser printer, print out some clip art, a cool digital scrapbook design, or your own custom artwork if you're tech-savvy. Cut out ten squares, about 1.5-2.5 inches or more, depending on your nail size. Apply base coat and two coats of white polish to your nails. Let them dry completely. Pour enough rubbing alcohol into a small cup or shot glass to cover your fingertip past the cuticle. Dip one finger in to the alcohol and count to five. Immediately press one of the squares onto your wet nail with the image face-down. Keep the paper very still and count to 20 while pressing down firmly. Then slowly peel off the square; you should see the image transferred onto the nail. Repeat with each nail and apply top coat.

✳ STORING YOUR LOOT

As you build your nail art skills, you may accumulate quite a stash of products and tools. Let's talk storage before your supplies get out of control!

STORAGE BINS

I use a tall chest to hold all my nail paraphernalia, but you may find that a large drawer, art bin, or tackle box works well for your needs. Bins with foldout trays are compact for travel and keep supplies easily accessible. If you outgrow your first storage bin, you can still use it to take a smaller selection of supplies on the road.

CLEAR ACRYLIC DRAWERS AND BINS

Clear acrylic boxes and bins with dividers are perfect for storing nail polish. You can also use them to store miscellaneous items like nail glue, treatments, gels, toe separators, dapping dishes, nail wheels, and dotters.

PENCIL CASES AND POUCHES

Soft pouches are great for storing metal tools because sharp items like nippers and tweezers can be damaged if they bump up against the sides of hard containers. Hard cases make a perfect home for emery boards, wood pushers, and buffers.

CRAFT BOXES

Transparent plastic crafting boxes have many small compartments to keep nail supplies well-organized and accessible. I use them to house all my crystals, studs, pearls, glitter jars, decals, and more.

BRUSH HOLDERS

I store my brushes in a brush holder that is designed to help them keep their shape. Brush holders are usually available at art supply stores.

ZIPPER STORAGE BAGS

Keep bottles of liquids like acetone in zipper storage bags to prevent spillage. Harsh chemicals are best stored in a bottom drawer below other valuable items to prevent damage from leaks.

CANISTERS

Lidded candy jars or toiletry canisters hold cotton balls, swabs, and pads with ease.

✳ MAINTAINING YOUR SUPPLIES

Here are some guidelines for keeping your supplies fresh, clean, and ready for use.

POLISH

Unopened bottles of lacquer can last up to a year and a half, and longer if stored properly. Keep your polish bottles in a cool, dark, dry place, as extreme temperatures and direct sunlight break down polish. Old or improperly stored polish will separate or become thick and gooey.

ACETONE AND OTHER REMOVERS

Nail polish remover and acetone are flammable and they should be stored away from heat, electrical outlets, and flames. Containers should be airtight to prevent evaporation and limit exposure to toxic fumes. Keep removers out of reach of children and pets.

METAL TOOLS

Pristine metal files, pushers, tweezers, and cuticle nippers are essential for proper nail grooming. Wash and dry tools after every use and lubricate any movable parts with cuticle oil to prevent rust. Store tools on their sides to keep them sharp; storing tools with the points facing down is a sure way to bend or dull them.

FILES, BUFFERS, AND WOODEN PUSHERS

These tools are porous and cannot be effectively cleaned, so replace them regularly. I recommend keeping used files, buffers, and pushers separate from new ones to avoid contamination. These tools should all be kept dry to prevent mold.

NAIL ART BRUSHES

Cleaning your brushes after every use is crucial; once paint hardens in the bristles, there's no turning back. Never store your brushes with the bristles down, and don't leave them soaking in water for an extended length of time, as they will lose their shapes and fray. Always dry your brushes fully before putting them away, and use brush caps to protect their shapes and to keep them dust-free. (You can purchase brush caps at any art store.)

LOTIONS, OILS, SCRUBS, AND TREATMENTS

Lotions, oils, scrubs, and treatments should be kept in a cool, dry place. Check expiration dates and use or discard as recommended by the manufacturer.

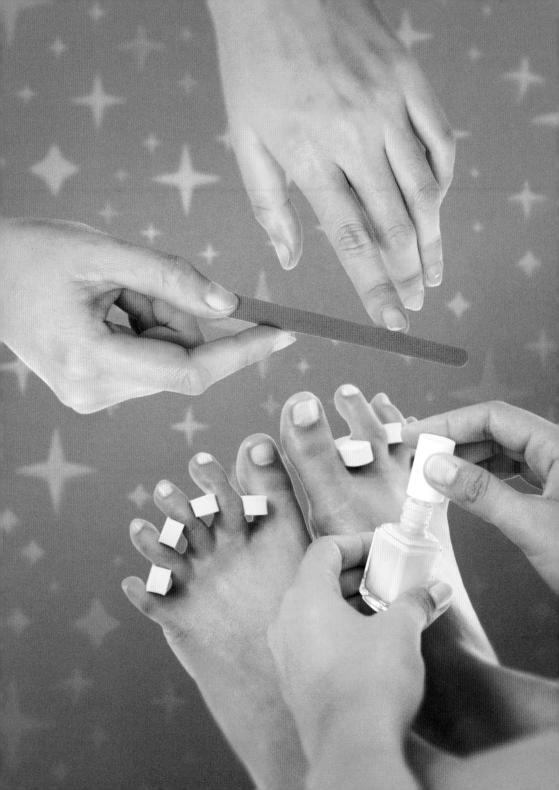

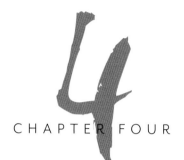

manicures and pedicures

Now that you're familiar with all the parts and players, it's time to get those fingers and toes in shape with a manicure and pedicure. In this chapter we will learn to set up what I like to call a "pop-up nail salon" at home. We'll cover how to choose the right nail shape and perfect it with polish so you can turn out a professional-looking nail service without stepping out your door.

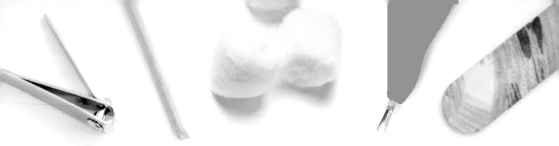

✳ SETTING UP FOR MANICURE

It's important to set up all the items you need before you start getting busy. Nothing is more annoying than stopping mid-manicure to run and get a buffer or bottle of top coat. Here's how to assemble a pop-up manicure and pedicure station like a pro.

1) Clean off your workstation. I like to use a snack tray, but if you don't have one, any flat, sturdy surface will do. Wipe down your area using the appropriate household cleaner for the surface you choose.

2) Make sure all your tools are clean. Of course, you are already cleaning and sanitizing your tools after every use, right? But I still like to give them a quick rinse to remove dust and other particles.

3) Grab something to put your trash in. Throughout your pampering, you will need to throw away cotton balls, wood pushers, paper towels, disposable files, buffers, and more. I prefer a small wastepaper basket with a lid to cover up any fumes from product, but you can always clip or tape a plastic bag on the side of your table. Just make sure you empty it after you're done.

4) Find a container to hold your used tools so they don't get mixed up with your clean ones. Storing them together will contaminate the cleaning tools. I like to use pencil boxes to keep my tools organized; one is just for clean tools and one just for dirty tools.

5) Place three paper towels or one hand towel (not too fluffy) in the middle of your workstation.

6) Place a finger bowl filled halfway with hot, soapy water in the middle of the towel. I like to set out hot water right away and let it cool while I finish setting up everything else.

7) Place the products you will be using on the edge of the table, on the side of your dominant hand. These products should include polish remover, cuticle remover, oil or moisturizers, base coat, top coat, and quick-dry.

8) Place the files, wooden pushers, and buffer between the products and the finger bowl.

9) Select a few potential polish colors and place them directly in front of you, behind the finger bowl along the edge of the table.

10) Place cotton balls or wipes next to the polish. I like to put them in a little dish.

11) Grab your tool boxes and place them on the side of the finger bowl opposite your products.

12) Place an extra towel or a few paper towels on your lap and grab a few extra towels or a roll of paper towels to have standing by, just in case you need them.

TOP TIPS FOR AN AT-HOME MANI-PEDI:

→ sterilize all reusable tools before use

→ prepare your station before you begin

→ allow plenty of time

→ file before soaking

→ polish your dominant hand first

→ let your polish dry completely

→ pamper yourself and enjoy the process!

SETTING UP FOR PEDICURE

1) Place a cloth towel on the floor. If you have a rug or carpet, lay a plastic bag down flat under the towel to prevent stains.

2) Put an empty basin on the floor, in the middle of the towel.

3) Grab a small end table, snack table, or firm ottoman.

4) Place all your tools on the table. I like to place the most-used items, like nail files, buffers, and wooden pusher, closest to me. Place products behind the tools, including lotion, polish remover, and callus remover.

5) Put your tool boxes on the table as well.

6) Add some nail polish colors, base coat, top coat, and quick-dry to the table.

7) Next to the basin, place foot files, flip-flops, toe separators, and a pumice stone.

8) Add soap, oils, botanicals, or other treatments to your basin.

9) Keep a number of extra towels on hand. Pedicures can get messy, so be prepared!

10) The last step is adding warm water to the basin. I like to use a water pitcher to slowly pour the water into the basin right before I start the pedicure. Don't try to carry a heavy basin full of hot water!

You can time your manicure and pedicure by your television! A basic mani should take the same amount of time as a sitcom, and a pedicure takes about as long as a drama. You should be able to complete a full mani-pedi while watching a feature film.

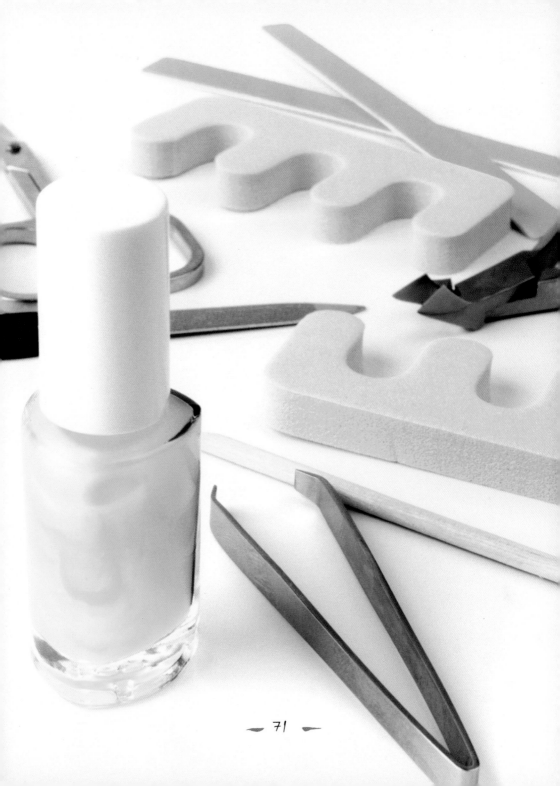

✳ PLANNING FOR TIME

The amount of time needed for a mani-pedi will vary based on previous nail care and skill level. Nails that have been primped and maintained on the regular will not take as long to treat as those that have been neglected. As the old saying goes, "practice makes perfect."

the manicure

A first-time manicurist will work more slowly and make more mistakes than a gal who has a long history of at-home primping. For beginners, a basic manicure can take anywhere from 45 minutes to an hour. Additional treatments and nail art will add extra time to the schedule. Your goal should be to get it down to 30 minutes:

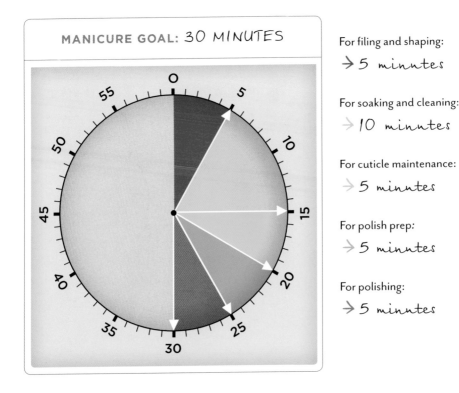

MANICURE GOAL: 30 MINUTES

For filing and shaping:
→ 5 minutes

For soaking and cleaning:
→ 10 minutes

For cuticle maintenance:
→ 5 minutes

For polish prep:
→ 5 minutes

For polishing:
→ 5 minutes

the pedicure

For beginners, a basic pedicure can take anywhere from 60 to 90 minutes. As with manicures, additional treatments and nail art will add extra time to the schedule. Your goal
should be to get it down to 45 minutes:

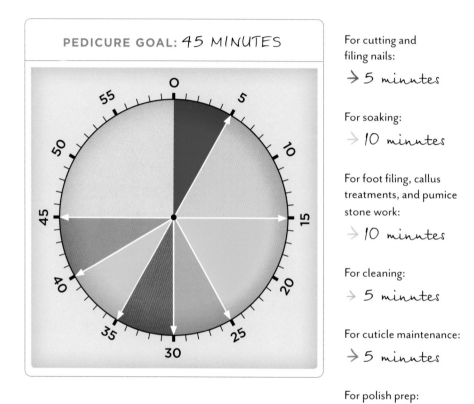

PEDICURE GOAL: 45 MINUTES

For cutting and
filing nails:

→ 5 minutes

For soaking:

→ 10 minutes

For foot filing, callus
treatments, and pumice
stone work:

→ 10 minutes

For cleaning:

→ 5 minutes

For cuticle maintenance:

→ 5 minutes

For polish prep:

→ 5 minutes

For polishing:

→ 5 minutes

Before you start polishing, make sure you have access to the things you usually reach for, like phones, wallets, and remote controls, so you don't damage your polish while digging around for them. Also try to make a trip to the ladies' room before applying lacquer; that's often where color gets ruined. When finished, make sure your nail polish is thoroughly dry before using your hands.

My favorite time to polish is right before bed. That way, you can paint and then go to sleep. You won't be tiptoeing awkwardly around, trying to avoid using your hands. Without a quick-dry product, lacquer can take 15 minutes up to a few hours to dry completely. Polish drying time also depends on the product you use. Every brand is different, but keep in mind that highly pigmented colors like deep reds and dark plums take longer to dry than light, sheer colors.

Give your polish a little time to settle in between each coat to help cut down on overall drying time. This will also make your polish less likely to chip and peel. Nail polish tends to take longer to dry in more humid weather, which is another reason I suggest polishing at night when temperatures are cooler.

✳ SHAPING THE NAIL

Modern ladies are, of course, free to wear their nails however they please. However, if you want to flatter your hands, here are some simple guidelines to follow. In general, the shape of the free edge should mirror the shape of the cuticle. This symmetry is the key to achieving the most delectable finished look. However, lifestyle is an important factor in selecting the best shape for your nails. Here's the rundown on picking the perfect shape for your pointers.

OVAL

It's hard to look bad in an oval nail. This shape flatters every finger, from narrow to wide, and always delivers a graceful look. Oval nails aren't the strongest or sturdiest, so you won't be doing manual labor while sporting these tips. To achieve this look, keep the sides of the free edge straight and slowly form the tip into an oval shape, making sure both sides are even.

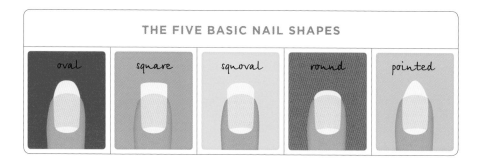

THE FIVE BASIC NAIL SHAPES

oval *square* *squoval* *round* *pointed*

SQUARE

Square nails are great for balancing out narrow fingers with longer nail beds. But beware: if your nail beds are short and wide, this shape will only make them look wider. To achieve this look, file the sides of the free edge straight up and down, and then file the tops straight across.

SQUOVAL

Squoval is without question the most popular nail shape. It combines the strength of the square shape with the elegance of the oval shape, giving you the best of both. To achieve this look, begin by creating the square shape, and then round the corner at a slight angle.

ROUND

Round nails are perfect for very active gals who like to keep their nails short. This shape works particularly well for those with long nail beds, but thicker fingers. To achieve this look, file the free edge in a half-circle from side wall to side wall.

POINTED

Pointed nails will make any hand look super skinny and a mile long. However, this shape tends to break and chip easily and lasts better on artificial tips. To achieve this look, evenly taper the sides of the free edge and bring them to a point at the tip.

NOTE: Square nails break more easily than round nails.

true confessions
of a luxury manicurist

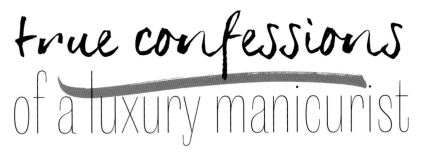

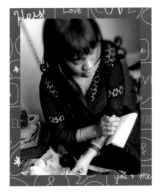

✳ On getting started as a luxury manicurist . . .

My journey as a luxury manicurist started in 2009 when I sought out and assisted a veteran nail technician in the industry. One day when I was assisting at a photo shoot for *Allure* magazine, the hair stylist on set informed me that her agency was looking for a manicurist. She gave me the agency's business card and I called as soon as I got home. The very next week, I was booked on a shoot for *Vogue Italia* and my name was printed in the credits.

✳ What draws me to nail art . . .

I've always been an artist and a fan of cosmetics. To me, the beauty industry has the power to transform a person inside as well as outside. I have a major fondness for makeup, and I spent time working solely as a makeup artist, but nails have always been my first love. I think it's because manicures and pedicures draw women together. There's something about a group of women getting together to have their nails done that is different from any other beauty service. You can easily talk to everyone around you (not just your stylist) and have amazing group discussions. I love a good girl-time powwow. Plus, with nails, the clients can enjoy my work just as much as the public. Clients can see their great haircut or banging makeup job only when they look in the mirror, but nail art is always in full view.

✳ On learning to perform manicures ...

I'm originally self-taught; I've been polishing as long as I can remember. My mother was also meticulous about her long, red nails, and my father could always be found grooming his nails in his spare time. As a kid at slumber parties, I was always the one breaking out the polish and lacquering everyone up! But I've now perfected my skills through beauty school and the guidance of mentors. When I graduated from nail school in 2009, I told my teacher that my work will be in magazines . . . and the rest is history.

✳ What I love most about nail art ...

I love the fact that clients can enjoy their nail art all the time, without the help of a mirror. I also love the staying power of nail art; it lasts longer than the cool makeup application you must regretfully wash off at the end of the night. But at the same time, nail art is not a big scary commitment, like an edgy haircut that takes time to grow out.

✳ On finding inspiration...

I get a lot of inspiration from textiles these days. It's easy to get lost in patterns, color schemes, and embroidery. I'm always eager to translate what I see in fabric stores onto nails. I also love to look at what's going on with nail art in Japan. Japanese nail art just looks so perfect; nail school is a big deal there. It takes many hours of training and tests to become a nail technician in Japan, and it shows in the work. Japanese nail artists can make highly detailed nail art with three-dimensional creatures, large rhinestones, and tons of glitter that somehow still looks dainty.

✳ On spotting the next hot nail trend ...

Nail art is so hot these days that any style you sport can be on-trend. Now I see more emphasis on nail health and a curiosity about how to cultivate truly healthy nails. I predict more interest in how a proper manicure service is performed, and the ingredients that are used in nail products. People who care about their nails are going to want to know what goes on behind the chair.

step-by-step
manicure

Okay, by now you should be sitting at your table, products and tools lined up, and a towel in your lap. LETS GO!

1) Removing Old Polish

Grab a cotton ball or wipe and saturate it with polish remover. Hold the cotton onto the nail and count to ten; this will give the remover time to eat through the old polish. Using light pressure, slide the cotton toward the free edge in a stroking motion. Repeat on all ten fingers until all traces of polish are gone. Always swipe away from you, and never into the cuticles or side walls.

2) Shaping Nails

Clip nails first, if needed. Select a desired nail shape and grab your file. Use a 180-grit board to file from one side of the free edge to the center. Then file from the opposite side to the center. Remember, you are not sawing down a tree, so don't drag the file roughly back and forth across your nails.

3) Soaking Nails

Soak filed nails in your finger bowl full of soapy, warm water, or try using water laced with oils and botanicals. The soaking process will loosen dirt and soften cuticles, making them easier to work with.

4) Cuticle Maintenance

After soaking, pat off excess water with a towel, and then dot on cuticle remover or cream. Use your wooden pusher to gently push your cuticles back. If you have excess skin tags, hangnails, or dead skin lifting off the nail plate, use nippers to cut them away. Don't use dull nippers that may pull or tear the skin. And remember, never cut living cuticle skin!

5) Cleaning and Drying

Now, grab your nail brush, dip it the finger bowl, and then brush your nails clean. Use the wooden pusher or cotton to nudge out any stubborn dirt. After this step, I suggest getting up and washing your hands. This is also a great time to wash your finger bowl. Dry your hands and nails using a towel. I prefer cloth, but paper towels will do. Make sure to dry between each finger.

6) Cuticle Oil

Next, dot on your cuticle oil. Use your thumb to massage the oil into your cuticle, trying your best not to get too much oil on the nail plate.

7) Buffing

Buff your nail plate with a nail buffer to smooth out its surface. Avoid using too much pressure. Buff the nail plate in an "X" pattern with downward strokes.

8) Applying Lotion

Massage your hands with lotion for added moisture and hydration (and super-soft hands!)

9) Cleaning the Work Station

Put everything away and clean up your mess now, so you won't run the risk of smudging your polish later.

10) Polish Prep

Grab a piece of remover-soaked cotton and use it to remove oil and lotion residue from the nail plate. Take your time and really get in there. Don't forget to clean under the free edge. This step will help to keep polish from peeling and chipping.

11) Polishing

There's a special technique to turning out a perfect polish.

→ First, grab your base coat.

→ Wipe most of the lacquer from the brush, leaving just a little bead on the tip of the brush.

→ Place the brush in the middle of your nail plate, one millimeter back from the cuticle.

→ With the lightest of pressure, glide the brush down the plate to the free edge.

→ Repeat on the left and right side. Use your thumb to pull down the side walls when painting next to them.

→ Cap off the edge of the nail by swiping the brush across the rim of the free edge.

Base coat dries pretty quickly; just wait about 60 seconds, then move on to the color polish. Apply your lacquer as described to the left, but use two coats instead of just one. Let these layers settle a bit, and then finish by applying one coat of top coat in the same fashion as described to the left.

12) Correcting Mistakes

Now you're almost done. Clean up any color that crept outside the edges of your nails over the side walls. Grab a wooden pusher and wrap a thin layer of cotton around the tip. Dip it in polish remover and wipe the stray polish away. I suggest wiping away polish errors after you have applied top coat.

tips and aftercare

→ Remember to keep your polish and your nails in tip-top shape; never use your nails as tools.

→ Oil your cuticles daily.

→ Always paint your dominant hand first. You may think painting with your nondominant hand is tricky, but just try doing it while your nails are wet.

→ Always polish from your pinkie to your thumb because your fingers tend to roll inward as you go.

→ Reapply top coat every other day to extend the life of your color.

→ Fix nicks right away. If you see a little nick, grab the color, patch it up, and seal it all together with another round of top coat.

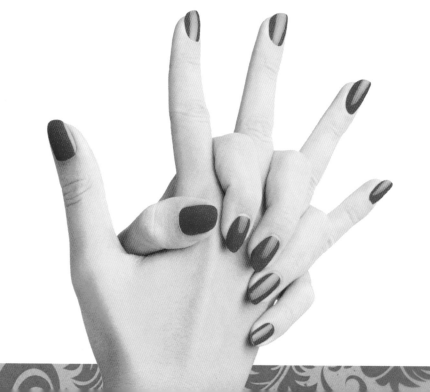

step-by-step
pedicure

Performing a pedicure is very similar to performing a mani-cure. As with a manicure, practice makes perfect. Practice weekly and your feet and toes will look simply gorgeous, darling.

1) Removing Old Polish

Grab a cotton ball or wipe and saturate it with polish remover. Hold the cotton onto the toenail and count to ten; this will give the remover time to eat through the old polish. Using light pressure, slide the cotton toward the free edge in a stroking motion. Repeat on all ten toes until all traces of polish are gone. Always swipe away from you, never into the cuticles or side walls.

2) Shaping Toenails

Trim toenails using a nail clipper, then file to smooth and shape. Use a 180-grit board to file from one side of the free edge to the center. Then file from the opposite side to the center. Remember, you are not sawing down a tree, so don't drag the file roughly back and forth across your nails. Be careful not to cut toenails too short, as that can lead to ingrown nails.

3) Soaking Toenails

Place both feet in the foot bath and soak for as long as you like. Take time to enjoy this step; turn on a movie or grab a magazine, and relax!

4) ## Cuticle and Callus Maintenance

After soaking, pat off excess water with a towel, and then dot on cuticle remover or cream. Let it sit while you use your foot file or pumice stone to soften dry, hard calluses from the heels, balls, and sides of feet, avoiding the toes and tops. Use your wood pusher to gently push your cuticles back. If you have excess skin tags, hangnails, or dead skin lifting off the nail plate, use nippers to cut them away. Don't use dull nippers that may pull or tear the skin. And remember, never cut living cuticle skin!

5) ## Cleaning and Drying

Dip your feet back into the bath and use a nail brush to clean them by scrubbings the tops, bottoms, and between your toes. Use the wood pusher or cotton to nudge out any stubborn dirt. Thoroughly dry your feet.

6) ## Applying Lotion

After all that hard work, it's time for a reward! Sit back down at your station, put a towel on the floor in front of you, and moisturize your feet. Take your time applying lotion or oil, using smooth, firm strokes to massage those sore muscles. Take the time to pamper yourself.

7) ## Cleaning the Work Station

Apply your toe separators and pedicure slippers. Dump your basin in the bathtub and clean up the messy remains on your workstation.

8) ## Polish Prep

Grab a piece of remover-soaked cotton and use it to remove oil and lotion residue from the nail plate. Take your time and really get in there. Don't forget to clean under the free edge. This step will help to keep polish from peeling and chipping.

9) Polishing

Use the same technique from the step-by-step manicure to turn out a perfect polish.

→ First, grab your base coat.

→ Wipe most of the lacquer from the brush, leaving just a little bead on the tip of the brush.

→ Place the brush in the middle of your toenail plate, one millimeter back from the cuticle.

→ With the lightest of pressure, glide the brush down the plate to the free edge.

→ Repeat on the left and right side. Use your thumb to pull down the side walls when painting next to them.

→ Cap off the edge of the toenail by swiping the brush across the rim of the free edge.

Wait about 60 seconds after applying base coat, then move on to the color polish. Apply two coats of lacquer as described above. Let these layers settle a bit, and then finish by applying one coat of top coat.

10) Correcting Mistakes

Now you're almost done. Clean up any color that crept outside the edges of your nails over the side walls. Grab a wooden pusher and wrap a thin layer of cotton around the tip. Dip it in polish remover and wipe the stray polish away.

tips and aftercare

→ File toenails straight across, or slightly round the corners. Be careful not to overfile the sides of the free edge, as that can lead to ingrown toenails.

→ Keep the floor around your pedicure area dry to avoid slipping on wet floors.

→ Try not to put on shoes for at least an hour after polishing.

→ Moisturize your feet daily.

→ Always wipe the bottoms of your feet after moisturizing, before sliding on your slippers, so you don't slip and fall.

→ If you experience foot problems or pain, make an appointment with your doctor.

→ If you have diabetes, check with your doctor before performing a pedicure at home.

✳ MEN'S MANICURE AND PEDICURE

Some fellas might think manicures are just for ladies, but I've got news for those dudes: good grooming cannot stop at the hands. Rough palms, overgrown cuticles, and jagged nails are a major turn-off. And I'm not just talking about turning off the ladies—raggedy nails will set you back in the professional world too. A little nail maintenance goes a long way. No need for polish; buffing is typically the method of choice for the well-groomed gent. Round nails are the most common, and more cuticle work is usually needed. To perform a men's manicure, follow each step as outlined on pages 78 to 80, but omit the polish and add some extra buffing as described below. Be aware that overbuffing can cause serious damage to your nails and the skin around them. Buff nails no more than twice per month to avoid damage.

Standard Buffer

Buff the nail plate with a standard nail buffer to smooth out its surface. Avoid using too much pressure. Buff the nail plate in an "X" pattern with downward strokes.

High-Shine Buffer

The high-shine buffer is a block or stick with different colored and textured surfaces for different types of buffing and smoothing. One section removes ridges, another section smooths the nail plate, and a third section buffs the nail to a super-high shine without any polish. Some stick-shaped buffers have an additional section for nail filing.

If you can use a standard buffer as described previously, using a high-shine buffer is not much more complicated. You can easily find high-shine buffers in most beauty supply stores. They typically have numbers printed on them; these numbers tell you the order in which you should use each section.

SIDE TWO: BUFF
Run this section along your
entire nail plate to buff
away ridges or peeling. Use
caution to avoid damaging
the nail.

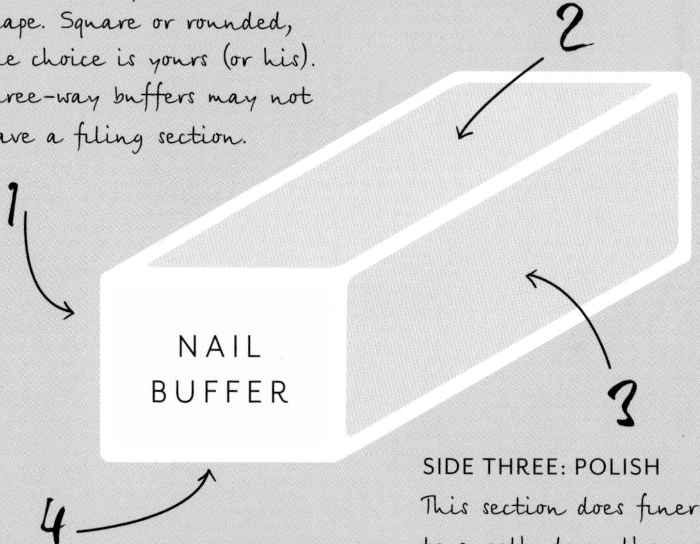

2

SIDE ONE: FILE
This section perfects the nail
shape. Square or rounded,
the choice is yours (or his).
Three-way buffers may not
have a filing section.

1

NAIL
BUFFER

4

3

SIDE FOUR: SHINE
This final step leaves a glossy
sheen on the nail plate.
After you see the shine you
get from buffing, you may
lose the urge to polish!

SIDE THREE: POLISH
This section does finer buffing
to smooth down the new nail
surface. This step will take
care of any tiny imperfections
missed during the buffing step.

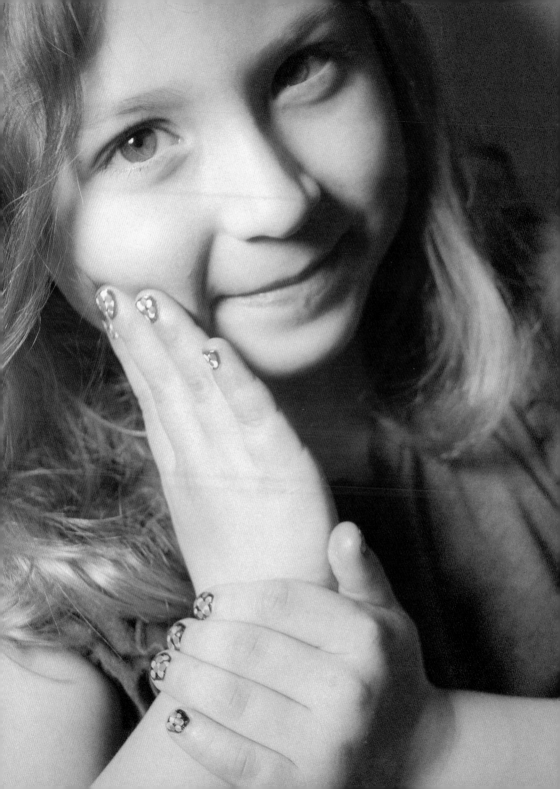

CHILDREN'S MANICURE AND PEDICURE

Little tykes love cute and colorful nails! Performing a mani-pedi on a child is a fun and creative activity, but take care when handling young paws and claws. Follow the basic manicure and pedicure as outlined on pages 78 to 80, using the following precautions to protect little hands and feet:

→ Children's nails are much softer than adults. Their nail plates have half the number of layers and are very pliable. Only use gentle, fine-grit files with very light pressure.

→ Set aside the nippers. Never cut the skin around children's nails! Their skins is very supple and it's hard to tell where blood vessels end.

→ Steer clear of hazardous products. Kids love to put their hands in their mouths, so only use nontoxic lacquer, lotion, and oil.

→ Little ones can be squirmy, so hand and foot baths may get messy. Clean their hands, nails, and feet with damp washcloths instead. Use a separate cloth for the hands and feet.

→ Help active tots wait for their nails to dry before digging for toys. Make a game out of protecting their polish by waving hands in the air in silly movements!

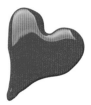

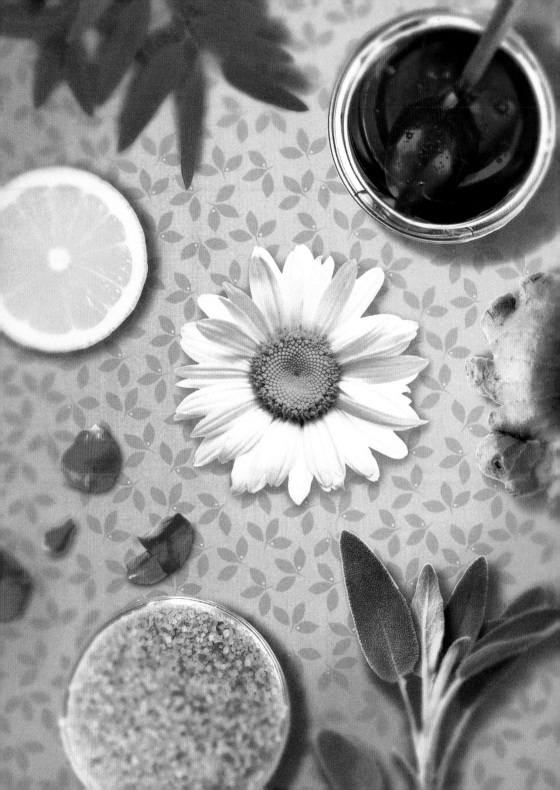

CHAPTER FIVE

beyond the basics

Now that you're a mani-pedi pro, let's kick it up a notch with some indulgent add-on treatments. Perks like botanicals, aromatherapy, and deep moisturizers can be the icing on the cake of your already-yummy experience. If you have the time for some extra luxuriating, use these treatments to take your manicures and pedicures to the next level of natural healing.

✳ BOTANICALS

Botanicals are beneficial ingredients derived from nature. If you've ever enjoyed a custom manicure or pedicure at a spa, you probably were treated with a variety of natural elements. Some of the best exfoliators are made of sea salt. Jojoba oil and shea butter are primary ingredients in most moisturizers. These products are naturally derived and have been used for centuries.

✳ AROMATHERAPY

Aromatherapy is the practice of using scents to stimulate the brain and body. Aromatherapy is used to relieve a host of physical and emotional conditions, including stress, pain, insomnia, low energy, and infection. Light candles or burn incense to fill the space around you with healing scents. Add fragrant oils to your finger bowl and pedicure tub to enjoy all the benefits that aromatherapy can offer.

✳ NATURAL INGREDIENTS AND THEIR USES

Lavender and Lavender Oil

Lavender has a calming and soothing effect. It also has anti-inflammatory and antimicrobial properties.

Lemon

The scent of lemon is invigorating. Incorporate lemon into your aromatherapy routine when you want to wake up or feel more energized. Lemon is also a stellar exfoliant for dry, flaky skin.

Chamomile

Chamomile soothes itchy, dry, sensitive skin.

Eucalyptus Oil

Eucalyptus stimulates blood circulation and acts as a pain reliever.

Ginger

Ginger is excellent for stimulating blood flow. The aroma of ginger is also stimulating and energizing.

Grapeseed Oil

Grapeseed oil is an amazing lightweight skin moisturizer. It's also excellent for reducing puffiness.

Mint

Peppermint and spearmint are both commonly used to rejuvenate tired, achy feet. The menthol scent relieves stuffy noses and alleviates stress. Mint is highly antibacterial, as well.

Olive Oil

Olive oil is an A+ moisturizer for hands and feet. Olive oil typically works well for people with allergies and sensitivities.

Honey

Honey is a humectant that helps the skin retain moisture and elasticity. It also has antioxidants that boost your body's natural defenses.

Heavy Cream

Heavy cream moisturizes and softens the skin, adding elasticity.

Jojoba Oil

Jojoba oil is an excellent moisturizer that fully penetrates the skin.

Bergamot Oil

The smell of bergamot has antidepressant qualities; use it to lift your spirits when you're feeling blue. Bergamot has antibacterial properties as well.

Sea Salt

Sea salt is an effective exfoliator for very dry skin.

Brown Sugar

Brown sugar is less abrasive than sea salt and can be used as a gentle exfoliator for sensitive skin.

Sage

Sage is naturally astringent and antiseptic. It kills the bacteria that cause body odor and controls excess oil secretion. Sage has also been known to regenerate skin cells.

Neem Oil

Neem oil relieves dry skin, itchiness, irritation, and redness. Neem oil is an effective natural treatment for psoriasis.

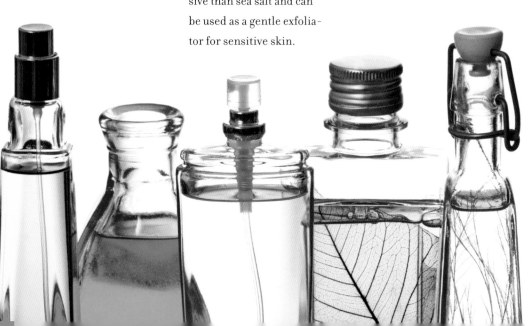

AROMATHERAPY TREATMENTS

Use the following recipes to create at-home aromatherapy treatments in your finger bowl or foot basin. The right aromatherapy treatment can offer instant relief for your ailments. Create your own unique combinations of the ingredients described on the previous page to blend custom aromatherapy treatments.

Lemon and Chamomile Nail Strengthener

1 chamomile tea bag
2 slices of lemon
1 tablespoon of olive oil
½ teaspoon of neem oil

Fill a pot with enough water to fill your finger bowl and bring to a boil. Remove from heat, add the tea bag, and let steep. Place lemon slices, olive oil, and neem oil in a finger bowl. Pour in the tea once it has cooled to a temperature comfortable for your hands. Soak your fingertips in the warm water for 15 minutes before proceeding with manicure.

Rose Petal Cuticle Hydrator

3 dried rose petals, crushed
½ cup of heavy cream
¼ teaspoon of honey
½ teaspoon of olive oil
1 ½ tablespoons of jojoba oil

Add rose petals, cream, honey, olive oil, and 1 tablespoon of the jojoba oil to your finger bowl. Fill with enough warm water to cover your fingers and soak for 15 minutes. Proceed with your manicure, but do not polish. Instead, use the remaining ½ tablespoon of jojoba oil and a soft cloth to buff your cuticles and nails.

Use these rules of thumb when developing your own treatments: in general, citrus scents are energizing, and floral scents are relaxing.

Invigorating Hand Exfoliator

¼ cup of brown sugar
¼ cup of olive oil
4 dried eucalyptus leaves
4 slices of fresh ginger
1 slice of lemon

Mix brown sugar, olive oil, and 2 crushed eucalyptus leaves in a small bowl and set aside. In your finger bowl, add the remaining eucalyptus leaves, ginger, lemon, and warm water. Soak for 15 minutes, and then proceed with your manicure. Before you prepare your nails for polishing, rub the brown sugar mixture on your hands for about 2-4 minutes. (Its best to do this over the sink.) Rinse hands and pat dry. Be sure to thoroughly prepare the nail plate for polishing by removing all traces of sugar and oil, and then proceed with polish.

Lavender and Mint Treatment for Swollen Feet

FOR FOOT BATH
3 bags of mint tea
1 cup of sea salt or Epsom salt
3 drops of lavender oil

FOR MASSAGE
5 drops of grapeseed oil

Fill a pot with enough water to fill your foot basin, and bring to a boil. Remove from heat, add the tea bags, and let steep. Place the salt and lavender oil in the foot basin. Pour in the tea once it has cooled to a temperature comfortable for your feet. Soak your feet in the warm water for up to 30 minutes. Pat feet dry, then massage with grapeseed oil before proceeding with pedicure. For added relief, elevate your swollen feet above your heart for 15 minutes.

Chamomile and Rose Treatment for Dry Feet

FOR FOOT BATH
2 bags of chamomile tea
½ cup of heavy cream
1 tablespoon of honey
3 drops of rose oil

FOR EXFOLIATION
½ cup of sea salt
¼ cup of coconut oil

FOR FOOT MASSAGE
½ teaspoon of jojoba oil

Fill a pot with enough water to fill your foot basin, and bring to a boil. Remove from heat, add the tea bags, and let steep. Place the cream, honey, and rose oil in the foot basin. Pour in the tea once it has cooled to a temperature comfortable for your feet. Soak your feet in the warm water for up to 30 minutes, then continue with pedicure.

After working on your cuticles, combine sea salt and coconut oil in a small bowl to make a scrub. Rub the salt scrub all over both feet for 2 minutes on each foot. Rinse your feet in the foot basin.

Pat feet dry, then massage them with jojoba oil before polishing.

Lavender and Tea Tree Oil Treatment for Sweaty Feet

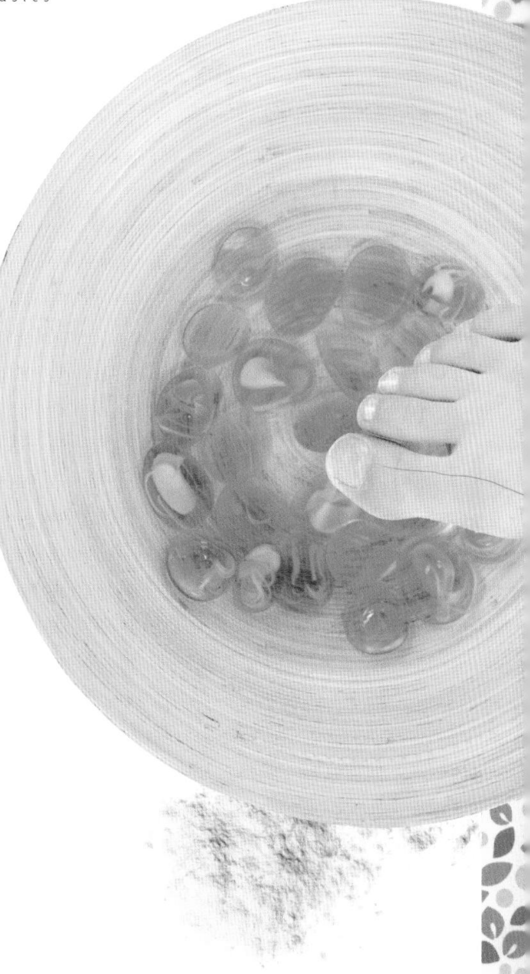

FOR FOOT BATH
2 bags of lavender tea
½ lemon, sliced
4 drops of tea tree oil

FOR FOOT MASSAGE
3 drops of sage oil
Baking powder

Fill a pot with enough water to fill your foot basin, and bring to a boil. Remove from heat, add the tea bags, and let steep. Place the lemon slices and oil in the foot basin. Pour in the tea once it has cooled to a temperature comfortable for your feet. Soak your feet in the warm water for up to 30 minutes.

Pat feet dry, then massage them with sage oil before polishing. After the polish dries, sprinkle feet with baking powder for added sweat absorption.

NOTE:
Gelatin powder is a secret fix for sweaty feet! Mixing gelatin powder with water in your foot basin works wonders for damp and sweaty feet.

✳ REFLEXOLOGY

Reflexology is the practice of massaging the hands and feet in specific areas where nerve ending are located, in order to bring relief to corresponding body parts according to reflexology maps.

Reflexology techniques vary and can involve using your thumbs, fingers, rubber balls, or wooden sticks to apply pressure. For safety reasons, reflexology is best performed by an experienced practitioner. However, if you want to obtain the benefits of gentle nerve stimulation at home, grab a friend or a partner and use the following charts to gently massage the hands and feet. Apply gentle pressure to desired reflexology points using your thumbs and/or forefingers. Use essential oils to add moisture, aromatherapy, and a smooth touch to your massage experience.

Reflexology requires repetition to reach its maximum potential, so keep practicing.

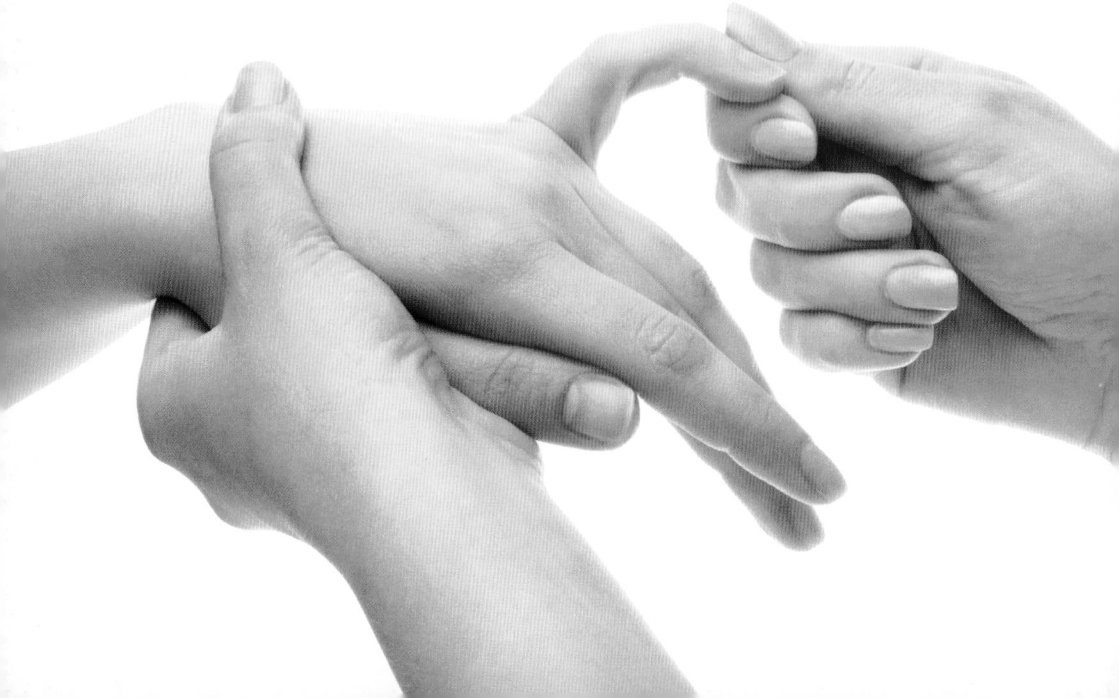

Remember that reflexology is not a cure-all, but it does provide helpful relief. Consult with a medical professional before using alternative therapies to treat medical conditions. Reflexology should be avoided or used with caution if you are pregnant in the first trimester or with high risk. It should also be avoided if you have epilepsy, cancer, diabetes, history of heart attack or stroke, and cuts, bruises, or sores on your extremities.

foot
reflexology
CHART

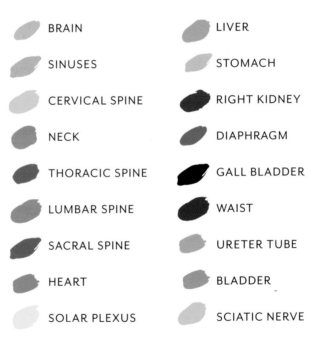

BRAIN

SINUSES

CERVICAL SPINE

NECK

THORACIC SPINE

LUMBAR SPINE

SACRAL SPINE

HEART

SOLAR PLEXUS

LIVER

STOMACH

RIGHT KIDNEY

DIAPHRAGM

GALL BLADDER

WAIST

URETER TUBE

BLADDER

SCIATIC NERVE

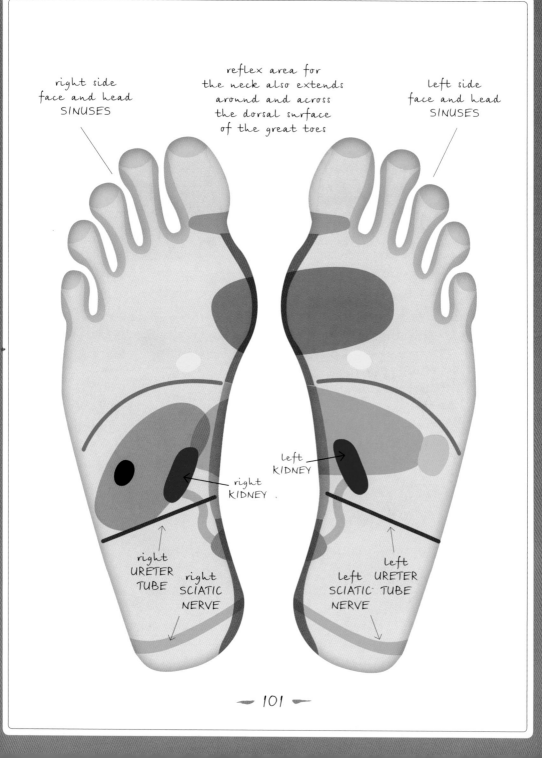

right side
face and head
SINUSES

reflex area for
the neck also extends
around and across
the dorsal surface
of the great toes

left side
face and head
SINUSES

left
KIDNEY

right
KIDNEY

right
URETER
TUBE

right
SCIATIC
NERVE

left
SCIATIC
NERVE

left
URETER
TUBE

hand
reflexology
CHART

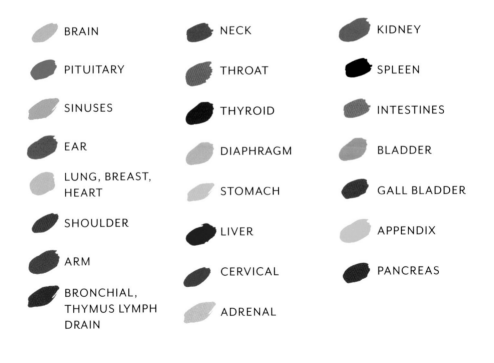

BRAIN

PITUITARY

SINUSES

EAR

LUNG, BREAST, HEART

SHOULDER

ARM

BRONCHIAL, THYMUS LYMPH DRAIN

NECK

THROAT

THYROID

DIAPHRAGM

STOMACH

LIVER

CERVICAL

ADRENAL

KIDNEY

SPLEEN

INTESTINES

BLADDER

GALL BLADDER

APPENDIX

PANCREAS

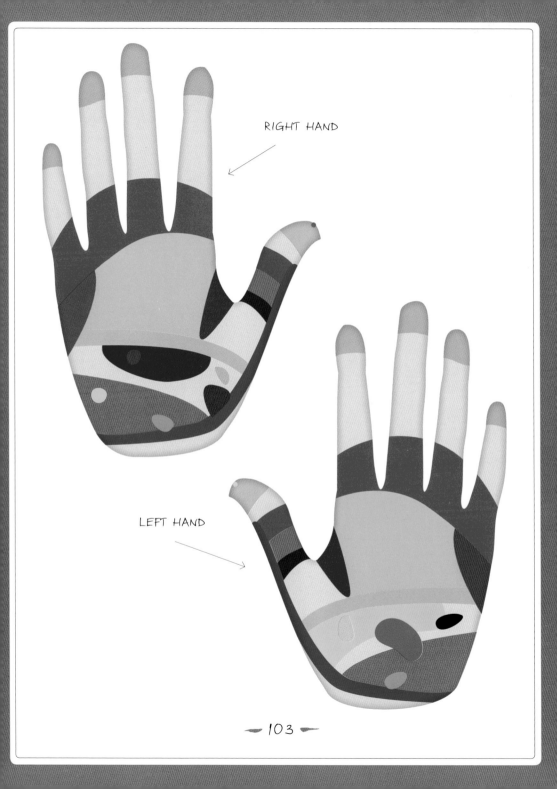

RIGHT HAND

LEFT HAND

PARAFFIN WAX TREATMENT

Give dry hands and feet an extra moisture boost with a paraffin wax treatment. This treatment uses heat to open pores and trap moisture in the skin. Paraffin wax treatments are especially helpful during the winter, when skin is most prone to dryness. They are also great for increasing blood circulation. Paraffin wax is typically white, odorless, and tasteless. It is used to make a variety of products, including candles, crayons, and wax paper.

To use paraffin wax as a moisturizing hand and foot treatment, heat the wax until it is melted and warm. You can also add a favorite aromatherapy scent to the melted wax. Slather your hand or foot with moisturizer and dip it into the wax to coat it. Once you pull your hand or foot out, you'll see the paraffin slowly harden and conform to the contours of your hand or foot as it cools. When cool, it will look and feel like a tight-fitting glove or sock.

At-home paraffin wax kits can be found in most beauty supply stores. Avoid double-dipping: repeat use of your paraffin wax unit will encourage the growth of bacteria and germs. Use these steps to keep it clean and safe for home use:

→ Three or more hours before your treatment, begin melting the wax in a pot on the stove. If you want to add some essential oils for aromatherapy, do so now.

→ When melted and warm, use a ladle to add one scoop of paraffin wax into a plastic bag.

→ Slide your hand or foot into the bag.

→ Spread the wax around your hand or foot.

→ Wrap a clean towel around the plastic bag.

→ Let the wax harden.

→ After about 10 minutes, slide the wax and bag off your hand or foot and discard.

→ Massage your hand or foot, wipe your nail plate, and continue with polish.

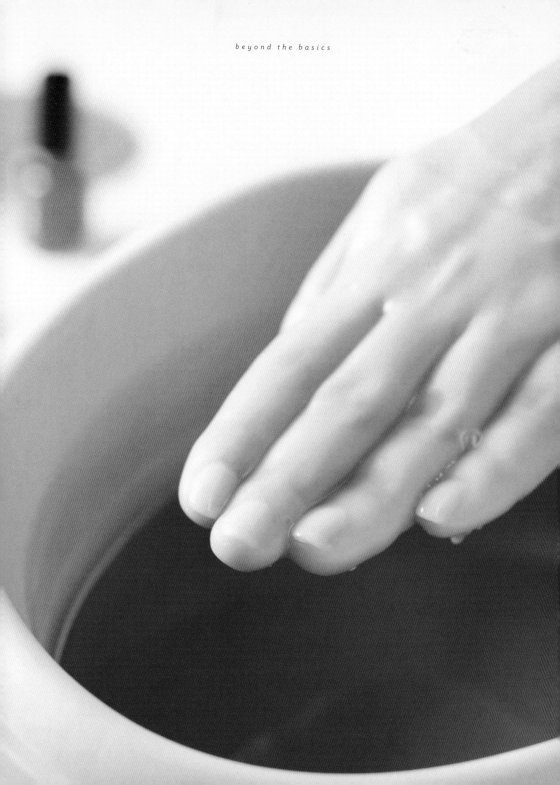

party time!

Throwing a mani-pedi party is the hottest new way to celebrate and pamper your friends. It's a great excuse for a female powwow, and you'll save yourself a trip to the salon. Here are some tips for hosting the perfect polish affair.

WHO'S WHO

Every party starts with a guest list. Aim for an even number of guests, as everyone will need to pair up. You might want to take a quick poll among your nearest and dearest friends to see who's available and down to polish. Remind your guests to save the date!

PICK YOUR PARTY STYLE

A truly stylish party always has a cohesive theme, design style, and color scheme. If your goal is to create a tranquil, spalike environment, go with flowers and soft, muted colors. For a movie-night manicure party, use black-and-white decor and play your favorite DVDs while you paint. Take inspiration from your favorite decade and look to the 1950s or 1980s for music, decor, and color choices.

YOU'RE INVITED

Sure, the quickest way to reach the gang is by text or e-mail. But think how cool it would be for your friends to open up a personalized invitation! A printed invitation sets the tone for your party; it is the gateway to an awesome event and gives your guest a sneak peek of the fun that's to come. Use your invitations as a canvas to creatively convey your party theme.

POLISH POTLUCK

Ask each guest to bring three to four favorite polish colors (and perhaps a small selection of nail art supplies). Remind your guests to skip their weekly manicures before your event.

PRE-GAME

Take some time to set up before your guests arrive. Make sure you have enough seating for every guest. For manicures, I like to use folding snack trays, but any table will do. Don't forget to put down a tablecloth! Pedicures can be performed anywhere from the couch to a folding chair. Set out large plastic tubs for pedicures, using one for every two people. Set aside a few small plastic bowls for manicures, and keep lots of extra towels on hand.

Put out a few bags of cotton balls, one or two bottles of cuticle remover and cuticle oil, and a couple bottles of polish remover so your guest can remove existing lacquer and clean up any manicure mistakes. I also like to keep a bottle of pure acetone handy for removing any particularly stubborn old polish.

Set out a few extra cuticle nippers and toenail clippers. It's nice to have one pair for each guest, but it's not necessary. If your guests will be sharing tools, you'll need a disinfectant like Barbicide and a soaking tray for cleaning metal tools between uses. Have plenty of wooden pushers, nail files, and buffers.

Lastly, set out a few different moisturizers and lotions. Scent is very personal, so aim for a variety of options and everyone will be pleased.

SET THE MOOD

Create a comfortable atmosphere so your guests can relax while their nails dry. Bring out big pillows, create a jammin' playlist, and prepare some tasty treats or order delivery. If you're of drinking age, find a great cocktail recipe or create your own! All that's left to do is to sit back and enjoy your company. Make it a night to remember.

SWAG BAG

Every great event has a parting gift. Pick up some inexpensive makeup bags from your favorite discount store and fill them with cute nail goodies like files, wooden pushers, top coat, polish, travel-size remover, and lotions. Now your guests can keep the party going at home.

pet PAWlish

Why should humans have all the fun? We pamper our pets in every way, and most of our furry friends are no strangers to bandanas and bows. Maybe you can't take your pet with you to the salon, but you can add a little color to their paws yourself at home.

You might be tempted to match your pet's polish to your own, but painting your furry friend with standard nail polish is a big mistake. Many nail polishes contain formaldehyde and other toxic ingredients that should not be ingested by animals who often put their paws in their mouths. Luckily, pet-safe lacquer and polish remover options are readily available. Now you can give your furry BFFs the manicures they deserve.

MY FAVORITE PET POLISH BRANDS:

→ Color Paw
→ Pawdicure Polish Pens
→ I ♥ Pet Head
→ OPI Pawlish

1) Make sure your pet is clean and fed. The best time to polish your pet's paws is after a meal when he or she is content and sleepy.

2) Take a good look at your pet's nails and make sure they're not cracked, split, or brittle. Do not paint damaged nails. If any nails have deep splits or cracks, they must be handled by a veterinarian. If there is just a tiny bit of cracking at the tip, you can easily sand it down with an 80-grit file or cut it with pet nail trimmers.

3) Sit on the floor, unscrew the polish bottle, and place your pet in your lap. Offer treats to keep your pet happy. When your pet is still,

quickly start painting. Work fast and don't worry about getting a perfect polish (just try not to get any polish on the fur).

4) Once all the nails are polished, you can let your pet run free, but keep frisky pets off of the furniture until the polish dries.

5) Enjoy your pretty pet as she struts her stuff. You'll be surprised to see how much some pets love to be polished.

6) When it's time to remove the polish, use the same tactics, with lots of treats to keep your pet calm.

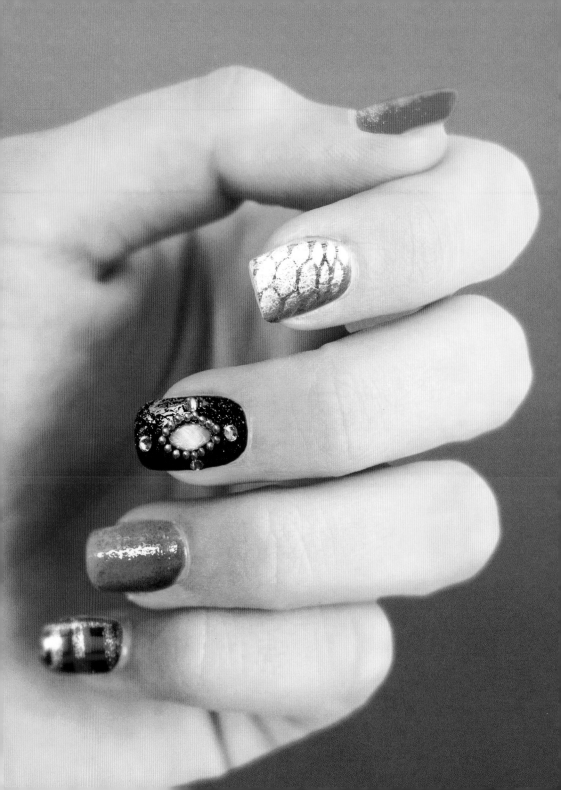

CHAPTER SIX

nail art

Don't fret if nail art looks like a difficult skill to master. Even Picasso had to start somewhere, and I guarantee that the place to start is the very beginning! In this chapter we will learn a few easy-peasy nail designs fit for the first-time nail artist. These tutorials will take you step by step through the basics, and by the time you're done, you'll have all the essential skills to be well on your way to becoming a spectacular nail artist. Let's begin!

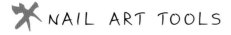

NAIL ART TOOLS

Nail Art Brushes

DETAIL BRUSHES
These brushes are designed to give you the most control. Their short, stiff, and fine tips make it possible to pull off the most intricate designs.

ANGLED BRUSHES
These brushes are great for painting borders, small to medium stripes, and fine strokes within your artwork.

STRIPER BRUSH
Use these brushes to create long, straight lines in one stroke. They are super easy to work with!

FLAT BRUSH
Flat brushes are great for filling in spaces like background areas or the white parts of French tips. They are best for short strokes.

FAN BRUSH
A fan brush is perfect for blending and layering colors. The fan brush also comes in handy when you want to remove dust or stray glitter.

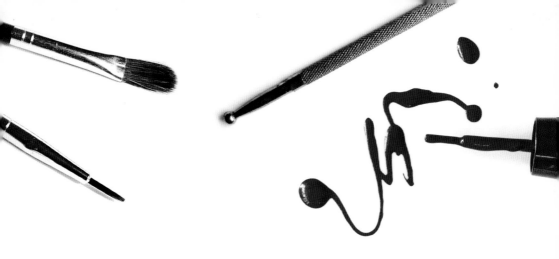

Nail Art Pens

The nail art pen is a new kid on the block. Like nail art polish, the pen makes it easer to create freehand nail art. These tools come in a push-pen form, with a marker-like tip and polish built into the body.

Dotter

This tool is great for making all sizes of dots on your nails. It works with polish or paint and can be substituted with a toothpick.

Nail Art Polish

These super-skinny bottles of nail polish come with a thin striper brush built right into the top. They are perfect for precise lacquer application, and great for freehand nail art designs.

Water-Based Acrylic Paint

Water-based acrylic paint is available at any craft store, and it is an amazing nail art tool. This heavily pigmented paint comes in a mind-boggling array of colors and can be applied to just about any surface, including nail polish and bare nails. Best of all, it can easily be removed with water, so if you make a mistake you don't have to remove your polish and start from scratch.

Painter's Tape

Painter's tape is available at any hardware store. I love to work with it because it's designed to cling to surfaces without becoming firmly attached. You can use it to create designs on your nails and then easily remove it without ruining your polish, unlike typical office supply tape.

dotted frames

A dotted design is the perfect starting place for experimenting with freehand nail art. The technique is basically "point and shoot." Follow these super-easy steps to sport a little dotted flash.

TOOLS

Base coat

Color polish or nail art polish in three to five colors

Top coat

Dotter or toothpick

1) Apply base coat and two coats of color polish, if desired. Unscrew the tops of all the bottles of polish, for easy access.

2) Using a small dotter and one polish color, make four dots along the perimeter of the nail plate: one at the top and bottom of the nail and one at each side.

3) Using another polish color, make four more dots along the perimeter of the nail plate, evenly spaced between the first dots.

4) Using a third color, make dots in the spaces between the first and second sets of dots. You can use a fourth color, if desired. Let the dots dry.

5) Apply top coat and let dry.

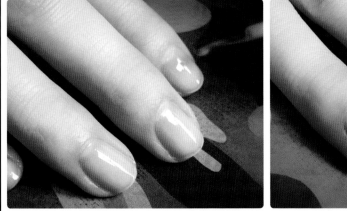

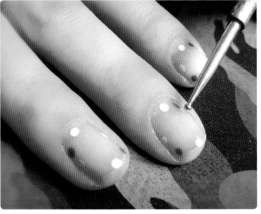

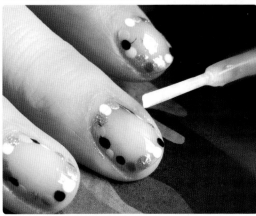

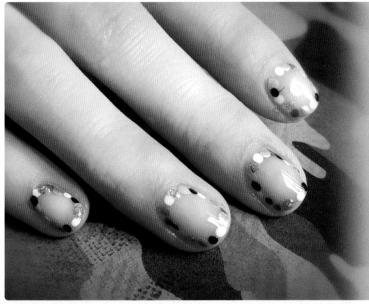

To make your nail art last, wipe the nail plate off with an alcohol-soaked cotton ball before painting.

flowers

Take your dotting technique to the next level with this floral design. Flowers have been the go-to nail art look since freehand nail design first came on the scene. What a great way to sport beautiful color and cheer any time of the year!

TOOLS

Base coat

Base polish color

A selection of complementary polish colors for flower petals

Yellow polish for flower centers

Top coat

Dotter

1) Apply base coat and two coats of base polish color. Let polish dry.

2) Grab your dotter and dip the tip in a petal color, taking care not to overload the dotter with too much polish.

3) Pick a spot on your nail plate (I like to start in the corner) and dot on five small dots in a circle, leaving the middle empty.

4) Repeat step three with a different polish color, as many times as you like, scattering flowers evenly across the nail plate.

5) Dip the dotter in the yellow polish and create a dot in the center of each flower.

6) Let dry and apply top coat.

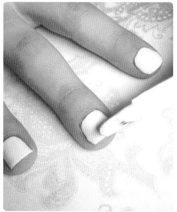
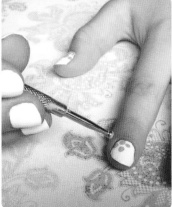
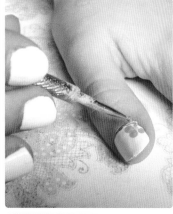
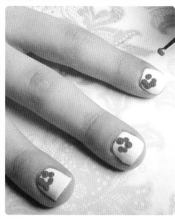
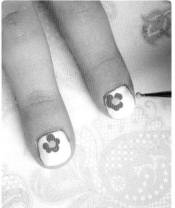
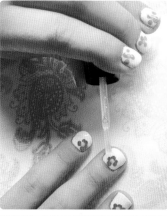
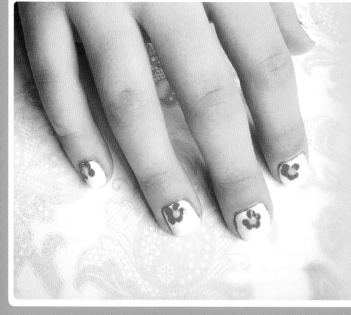

Flowers don't
have to be girly
and sweet.
If you're feeling
moody, go gothic
with your flowers
and choose deep
reds, purples,
and black.

pretty polka dots

Dots on top of dots on top of dots! This super-fun and easy design is guaranteed to draw admirers.

TOOLS

Base coat

Color polish in three to four shades that range from light to dark

Top coat

Dotter or toothpick

1) Apply base coat and two coats of base color polish, if desired.

2) Using a dotter and the lightest shade, paint dots starting from the free edge one-third of the way up toward the cuticle. Wipe the dotter clean.

3) Using the dotter and the medium shade, continue painting dots going up the middle third of the nail plate. Wipe the dotter clean.

4) Using the dotter and the darkest shade, continue painting dots going up the remaining third of the nail plate to the cuticle.

5) Let dry and apply top coat.

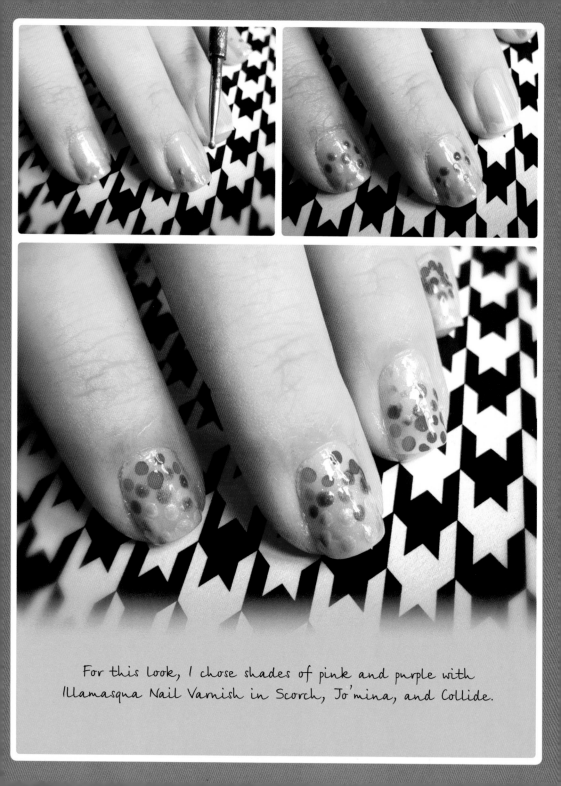

For this look, I chose shades of pink and purple with Illamasqna Nail Varnish in Scorch, Jo'mina, and Collide.

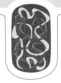

jackson pollock

Nail art or fine art? Your nails may look like they belong on a gallery wall, but this design is simple to execute and utterly mistake-proof. The best thing about this design is that you never get the same outcome twice!

TOOLS

Base coat

Two or more polish colors

Top coat

Dotter or toothpick

1) Apply base coat and let dry. Dip dotter or toothpick in one color and apply multiple dots all over the nail plate. Quickly wipe the dotter or toothpick clean.

2) Repeat step two with each polish color, working quickly so the polish doesn't dry.

3) Quickly swirl the dotter or toothpick around the nail plate in small circles until you develop a design you like.

4) Let polish dry and apply top coat.

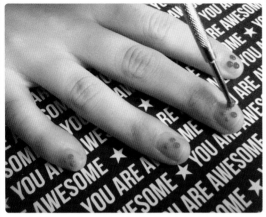
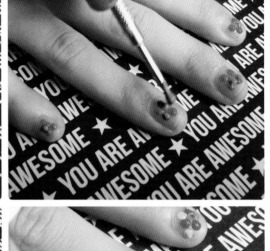
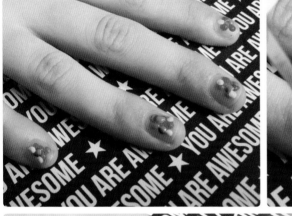
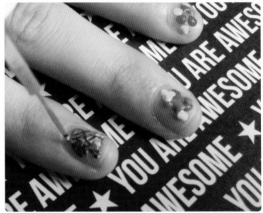
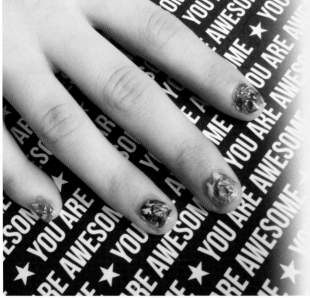

This design lets you go wild with color! Here I'm using a variety of primary colors, in the style of a Jackson Pollock painting. You can also experiment with varying shades in the same color family, or any of your favorite colors.

leopard print

Leopard print is defiantly wild and bold, but it's also classic and timeless. And that's the appeal! This pattern is downright sexy and not for the faint of heart. But hey, a little feistiness never hurt anyone.

TOOLS

Base coat

Base polish color

Two additional polish colors for leopard spots

Top coat

Dotter or nail art brush

1) Apply base coat and two coats of base polish color. Let polish dry.

2) Using one polish color and a dotter or nail art brush, paint squiggly half-circles, evenly spaced across the nail plate. Vary the direction of each half-circle for a more natural look.

2) Using the other polish color, create a messy dot in the center of each half-circle, covering most, but not all, of the half-circle.

4) Let polish dry completely and apply top coat.

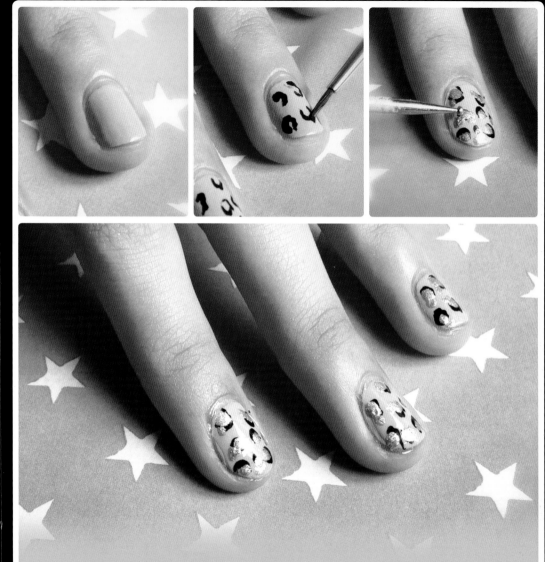

For a traditional leopard print design, stick to neutral shades. When you want a wilder look, get creative with your color schemes. Experiment with bright colors in complementary shades, but always keep some black or white in the mix to keep your design focused.

camouflage

The traditional military design was created to blend in with its surroundings, but this nail art design will most definitely stand out!

TOOLS

Base coat

Base color polish in army green

Nail art polish in black and two shades of green

Top coat

1) Apply base coat and two coats of color polish in army green. Let dry.

2) Apply the darker green shade in a few horizontal blobs, traveling from the side wall across the nail plate.

3) Apply the lighter green shade in varied squiggly horizontal lines.

4) Repeat with black nail art polish.

5) Apply top coat and let dry.

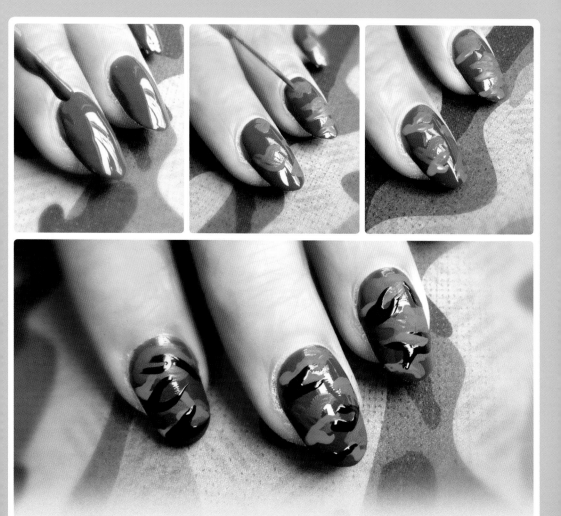

For this look, I'm using Illamasqua Nail Varnish in Rampage and Scorn. But don't limit yourself to the traditional army green! Try this camo design in your favorite colors for a unique twist on the original.

Here are some color combos to try:
* Army green, sage green, copper, and mauve
* Light blue, dark blue, black, and gray

ombré

The ombré trend is everywhere, from dip-dyed clothes to hair color, and now to your nails.

TOOLS

Base coat

Three to four polishes in different tints of the same color

Top coat

Makeup wedge sponge

Paper towel

Polish remover

Cotton swab

1) Apply base coat and let dry. Line the polishes up in order from lightest to darkest. Grab a makeup wedge sponge and lightly dampen it with water.

2) Take the lightest or darkest polish and apply a stripe of color along the thin end of the wedge. Alongside it, quickly apply a stripe of the next color in the line. Repeat with additional stripes from each polish color.

3) Dab the sponge on a paper towel a few times to blend the colors.

4) Line the tip of the wedge up with your free edge and firmly press it down on the nail plate like you're stamping it on. Dab the sponge in the same spot a few times (but try not to move it around too much).

5) Repeat steps four through seven for each nail.

6) Clean up any excess polish on your skin with a cotton swab soaked in polish remover.

7) Let dry completely and apply top coat.

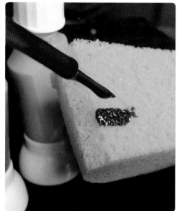 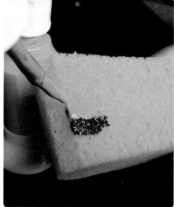 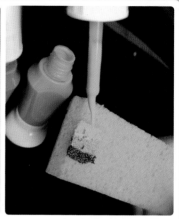

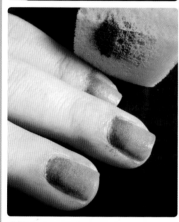 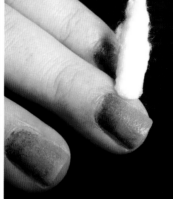 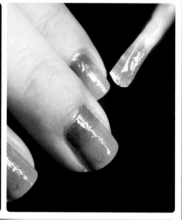

Take inspiration from color gradations found in nature. Evoke the ocean with blues and greens, or the sky with varying shades of blue.

pearly net

I love to experiment with unconventional items and tools when designing nails. The outcomes are always interesting! Try this tutorial using mesh fabric to get "How did you do that?" nails.

TOOLS

Base coat

Color polish

Top coat

Water-based acrylic paint

Netting or mesh fabric

Makeup wedge sponge

1) Apply base coat and two coats of color polish. Let dry. Cut a small piece of netting or mesh fabric, larger than your nail plate.

2) Dampen a makeup wedge sponge and cover it with a layer of water-based acrylic paint.

3) Place the netting or mesh fabric over one nail. Hold it steady by pinching it down with your fingers.

4) With the net in place, gently press the sponge over the nail plate to apply the acrylic paint.

5) Lift the net off and allow the paint to dry.

6) Apply top coat and let dry.

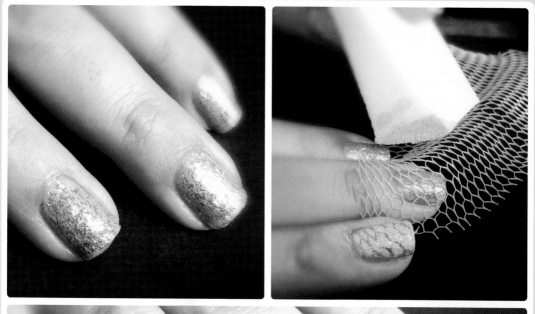

You can buy netting or mesh fabric from any craft or fabric store, but you can also get creative with items found around the house! Try using the mesh from a hair net or netting from a produce bag.

galaxy

Since the beginning of time, artists have been inspired to re-create the vibrant colors and spectrum of light above. The galaxy has an undeniable cosmic allure, and it's also downright cool! You may be thinking this design will take light years to create, but it's actually pretty easy. Follow these steps and you'll be riding the Milky Way before you know it!

TOOLS

Base coat

Color polish in black or dark blue

Glitter top coat

Water-based acrylic paint in varying colors, such as white, blue, purple, yellow, red, green, and pink

Wedge makeup sponges, cut in half and dampened with water

Paper towel

1) Apply base coat and two coats of black or dark blue polish. Let dry.

2) Drip a little bit of the lighter paint colors onto a paper towel on your work surface.

3) Dab the sponge into the paint and lightly sponge the colors onto the nail plate, one by one, taking care not to completely cover any color.

4) Repeat steps two and three with the richer colors. (I also like to sponge on a little metallic color for an added pop.) Let all the layers of paint dry.

5) Apply glitter top coat and let dry.

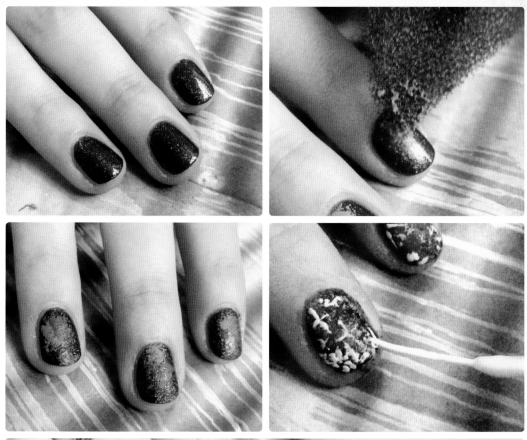

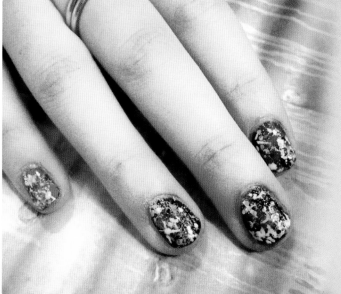

My favorite paint colors for this look are purple, pink, blue, gold, green, and burgundy. Experiment with different colors and find your own favorites!

vintage jewels

In this glamorous design, gold decals accent your tips like a piece of vintage jewelry. A few simple steps are all it takes to create this elegant look.

TOOLS

Base coat

Color polish

Top coat

Nail decals

Tweezers

1) Apply base coat and two coats of color polish. Let dry.

2) Using tweezers, peel off the sticker decals and place them on the nails wherever you like.

3) Press the decals into place and apply top coat.

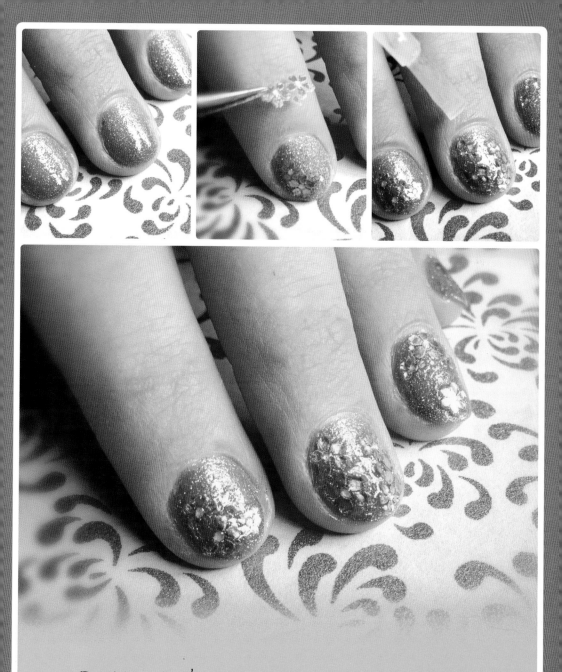

For this look, I'm pairing gold with purple and using
Zoya Nail Polish in Stevie, a sparkly violet shade.

neon sparkle

Neon = Cool.
Rhinestones = Cool.
Neon + Rhinestones = Super Cool.
Here's how to turn out this eye-popping design.

TOOLS

Base coat

Color polish

Glitter top coat

Clear top coat

Swarovski crystals in various colors, and in sizes 1.00 mm, 1.70 mm, and 2.00 mm

Tweezers

Wooden pusher

1) Apply base coat and two coats of color polish.

2) Apply one coat of clear glitter top coat.

3) While the top coat is still wet, use tweezers to pick up the larger rhinestones and place them on the nail.

4) Working quickly to keep the top coat wet, use your tweezers to pick up and place smaller rhinestones around the larger ones, creating clusters of stones.

5) Using a wooden pusher, secure the stones by gently pressing them into place.

6) Apply clear top coat around the stones and over the painted portion of the nail plate. Let dry.

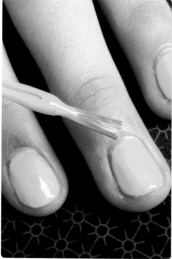 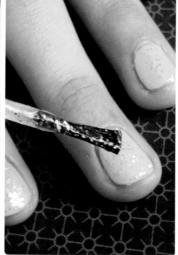 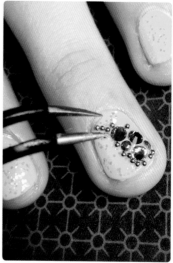

Think of this eye-catching rhinestone cluster like a special piece of jewelry, and wear it on just one accent nail.

When using rhinestones, don't apply top coat over the stones or it will dull their glimmer!

modern french

It's always fun to challenge traditions. Lets do just that by taking a plain old French manicure and turning it up a notch!

TOOLS

Base coat

Base color polish (optional)

Vibrant tip color

Black nail art polish

Flat nail art brush

Acetone

Dotter or toothpick

1) Apply base coat and two coats of base color polish, if desired. Let dry.

2) Paint the vibrant tip color across the free edge of each nail.

3) Dampen a small flat nail art brush with acetone and use it to clean up and even out your French tip.

4) Using a dotter and black nail art polish, apply polka dots on an accent nail. You can apply the dots randomly or in a pattern.

5) Let dry and apply top coat.

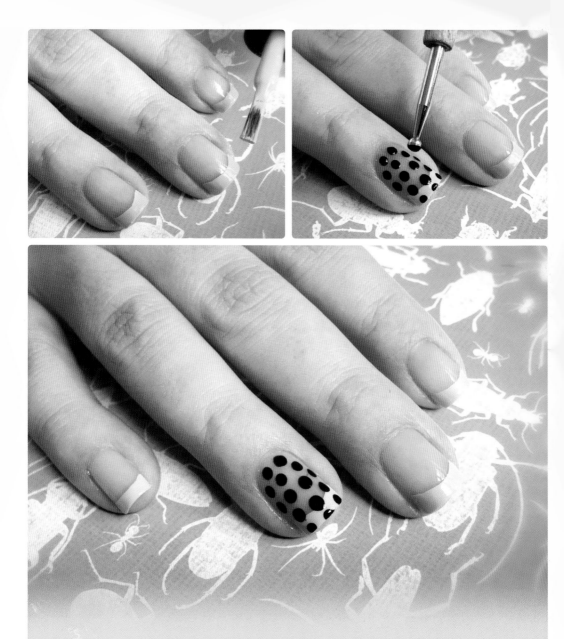

To ensure a perfect French tip every time, put tape on
the bottom half of your nail before painting.

rainbow bright

Traditional style gets so boring, and color is the spice of life! Why go for plain white tips with your French mani, when you can pump up the volume with bold hues and a touch of sparkle?

TOOLS

Base coat

Color polish in five complimentary colors

Glitter nail art polish

Top coat

Crystals

Tweezers

1) Apply base coat and two coats of color polish, painting each nail a different color. Let dry.

2) Using glitter nail art polish, apply a thin line across the tip of the free edge.

3) Apply top coat. While the top coat is still wet and tacky, use tweezers to apply crystals in various spots on the nail plate.

4) Let dry completely.

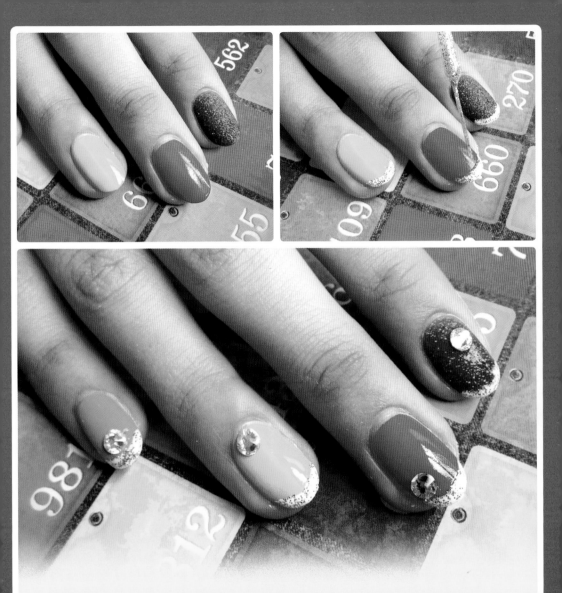

Here's a secret: you can use gems and studs to cover up any polish or nail art mistakes, and no one will be the wiser! In this look, the gems are placed randomly to add variety and interest. Work that to your advantage, and apply your stones wherever you need to hide a mistake.

crosshatch

This design is a bit uneven, so it looks natural and handmade. Channel your inner artisan and create a basketweave design on your nails!

TOOLS

Base coat

Nail art polish in three to four complimentary colors

Top coat

1) Apply base coat and let dry.

2) Using one color of nail art polish, paint a series of vertical and horizontal lines scattered across the nail plate. Go for crisscrossing lines in a "t" shape.

3) Repeat with each nail art polish color until you have filled the whole nail plate.

4) Let dry and apply top coat.

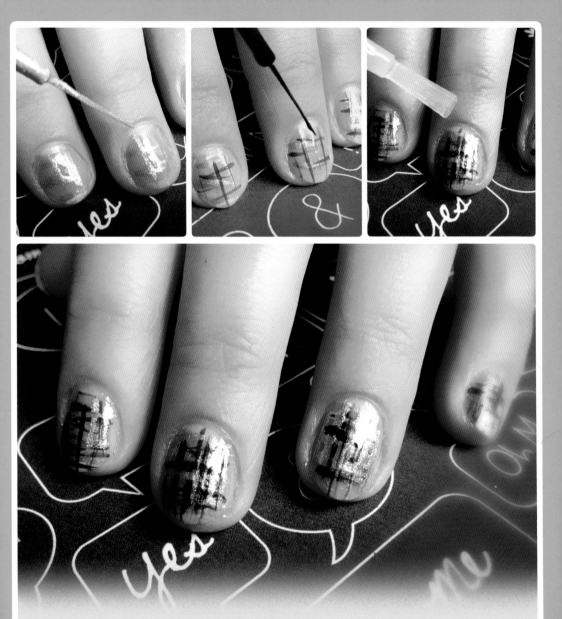

For this look, I used a shimmery neutral with shades
of black and blue to give it a little edge.

zebra print

In the wild, zebra stripes act as camouflage, preventing colorblind jungle cats from telling the zebra from the grass. But if you sport this chic pattern on your nails, you'll hardly blend in.

TOOLS

Base coat

Base polish color

Polish color for zebra stripes

Top coat

Striper brush

1) Apply base coat and two coats of base polish color. Let polish dry.

2) Using a striper brush, apply uneven stripes, both long and short, horizontally across the nail plate. Make a few stripes split off at the ends, like veins or branches.

3) Let dry and apply top coat.

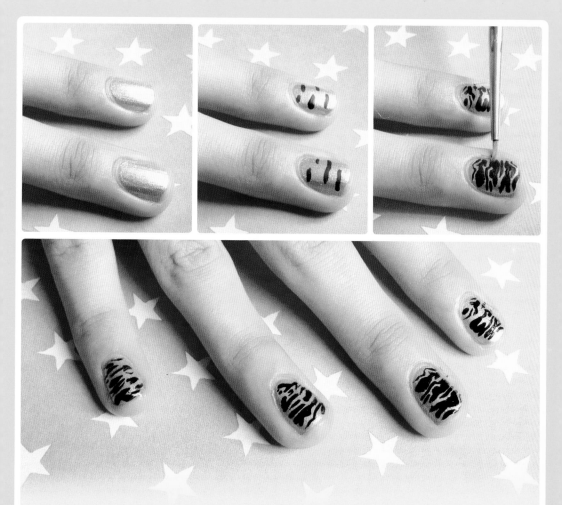

Don't limit yourself to black and white! Zebra stripes look killer in any color. But no matter what color combination you choose, paint the stripes the darkest shade.

Try these color combos:
* Hot pink and black
* Aqua and dark brown
* Lilac and charcoal
* Blush and copper

lightning bolt

The marvelous thunder and lightning storm is one of the most beautiful spectacles nature has to offer. Follow this easy tutorial and your nails will be just as spectacular!

TOOLS

Base coat

Color polish in dark blue or black

Nail art polish in white

Water-based acrylic paint in blue, purple, and white

Top coat

Makeup wedge sponge

1) Apply base coat and two coats of color polish.

2) Using the narrow tip of a makeup wedge sponge, apply a small amount of blue acrylic paint on the area closest to the cuticles. Repeat with purple paint, then white paint.

3) Using white nail art polish, paint wiggly lines resembling veins.

4) Sponge a little more acrylic paint over the lines to add dimension.

5) Let dry and apply top coat.

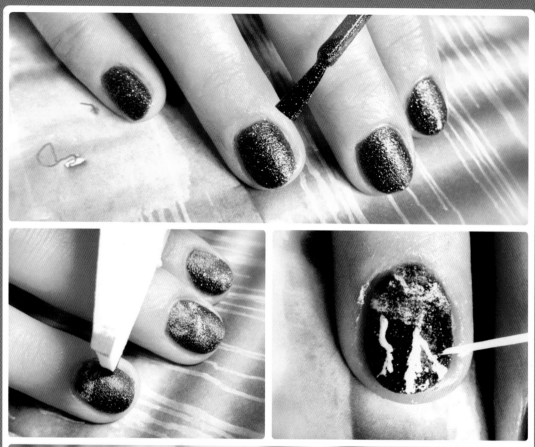

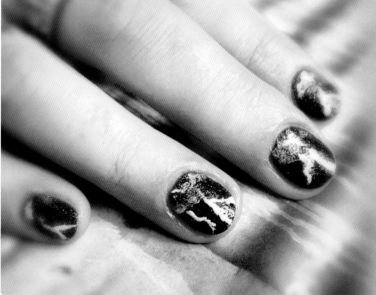

For this look, I'm using a shimmery black glitter color as a base color. You can also try a sparkly navy blue, like OPI polish in Yoga-Ta Get This Blue!

zigzag swag

Zigzag and chevron designs are trendy, striking, and—guess what—super easy to create! Use these tips to achieve a perfect zig and zag, every time.

TOOLS

Base coat

Base color polish

Nail art polish

Top coat

Dotter or toothpick

Striper brush

1) Apply base coat and two coats of base color polish, if desired.

2) Using a dotter or toothpick and your second polish color, paint two rows of stacked dots. The bottom row of dots should fall in between the top row of dots, as shown.

3) Using a striper brush and the same color polish, connect the dots, alternating between upper and lower dots to create a zigzag line.

4) Let dry and apply top coat.

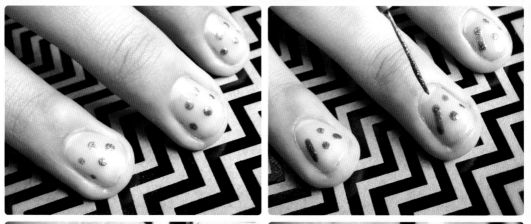

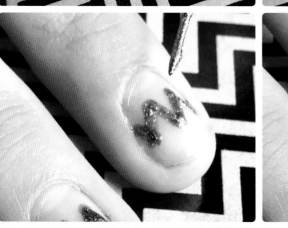

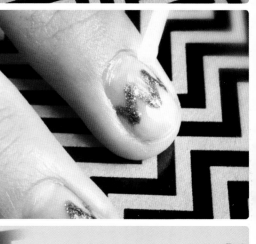

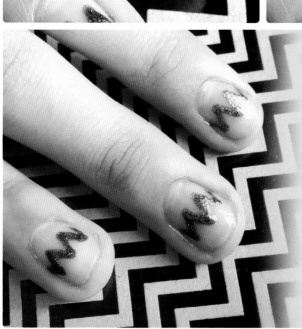

Still messy when it comes to your polish-ing skills? Try wiping a thin coat of white school glue on the skin around your nail bed and let it dry before applying lacquer to your tips. After painting, peel off the glue and the wayward polish will come with it.

hearts

No symbol represents passion and romance more than the heart. But to me, a heart also represents pure girliness! My junior high notebooks were filled with hearts—I even dotted my "i"s with hearts! So let's paint our nails with this iconic symbol; spreading love never looked so cool.

TOOLS

Base coat

Color polish

Top coat

Water-based acrylic paint in two colors

Angled brush

Dotter

1) Apply base coat and two coats of color polish. Let dry.

2) Using a dotter and acrylic paint, create two large dots right next to each other, anywhere on your nail.

3) Using a small angled brush and the same color paint, create a diagonal line from the outside of each dot to form a "V" shape.

4) Fill in the "V" and smooth out any rough edges.

5) Let dry and apply top coat.

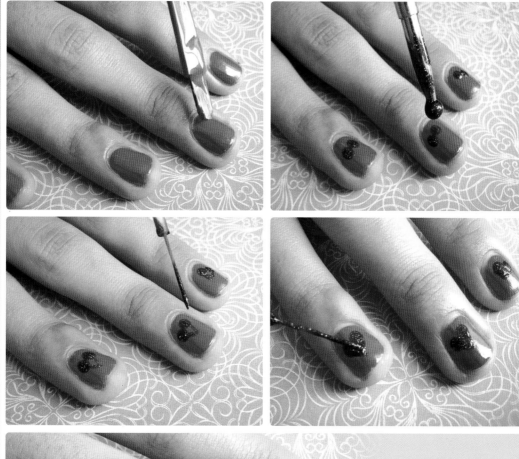

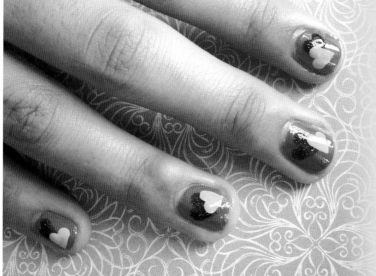

Be careful not to over-load your dotting tool with too much paint. Remember, less is more!

bow

Bows in our hair and on our clothing express a flirty girl-ishness. Paint one or two on your nails for the same effect!

TOOLS

Base coat

Base polish color

Top coat

One to two shades of water-based acrylic paint

Dotter

Detail brush

1) Apply base coat and two coats of base polish color. Let polish dry.

2) Choose an acrylic paint color and dip your dotter in it.

3) Begin your bow by dotting one large circle anywhere on the nail plate, making sure to leave room on either side.

4) Using a smaller dotter, build a bow by first poking two small circles on each side of the big middle one.

5) Before the smaller dots have time to dry, gently drag each toward the center of the large circle on a slight angle, like you're making a triangle. Paint small tails extending from the center of the bow.

6) Let the design dry a bit. If you like, outline your bow in another color (I like to use black) by making a thin line around the edges with a detail brush.

7) Let the design dry completely and apply top coat.

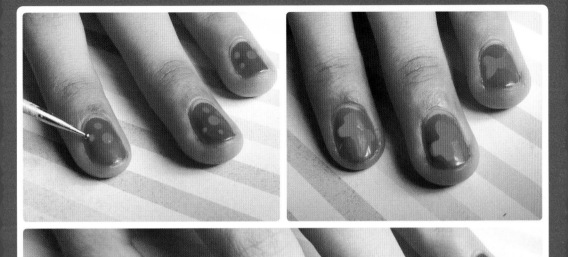

In this design, I used tonal shades for a subtle look.
If you want your bow to pop, work with complementary
shades. Paint a pale aqua bow on a coral nail, or a
bright yellow bow on a violet nail.

Polish dries faster with hot air, so if you're in a hurry,
plug in your hair dryer, set it to low, and aim it
at those wet tips. Keep the dryer moving so you don't
burn yourself.

music notes

Hit some high notes with this design, perfect for a music-loving chick who can't keep her favorite tunes out of her head. Now you won't be able to keep your favorite notes off your fingers.

TOOLS

Base coat

Base polish color

Top coat

Water-based acrylic paint in black and white

Striper brush

Detail brush

Dotter

1) Apply base coat and one coat of base color polish. Let dry.

2) Begin painting music notes by using a dotter and making three slightly oval-shaped circles. Paint two circles close together and one a bit apart from the other two.

3) Using a short, firm detail brush, paint a stem on the right side of each circle.

4) Connect the two notes that are closest, with one horizontal line at the top of the stems. Add a small tail to the other note.

5) To make the design pop and to create dimension, try to outline a few areas on the notes in white. This will really make you look like a pro!

6) Let paint dry and apply top coat.

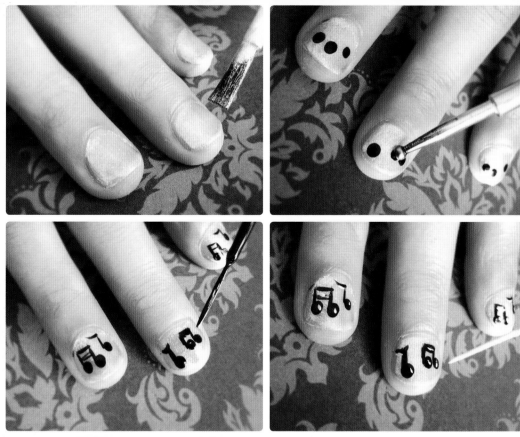

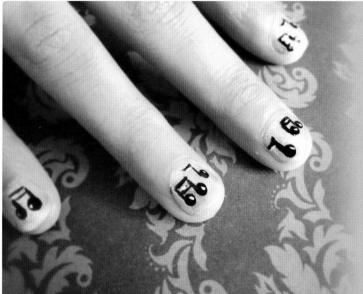

For this look,
I'm using
Silver Sweep by
Sally Hansen
Insta-Dri Flash
Dry Nail Color.

checkered print

While this print looks intimidating, it's actually very easy to pull off, and the finished look is incredibly chic.

TOOLS

Base coat

Base color polish

Top coat

Water-based acrylic paint in white or a complementary shade

Striper brush

1) Apply base coat and two coats of color polish. Let dry.

2) Using a striper brush and water-based acrylic paint, paint evenly spaced vertical stripes from the top of the nail all the way to the bottom. Let dry.

3) Using a clean striper brush and your base color polish, paint another set of evenly spaced stripes, horizontally from left to right across the whole nail.

4) Fill in the corner and center squares.

5) When done, you should have nails that resemble a checker or chess board. Let dry and apply top coat.

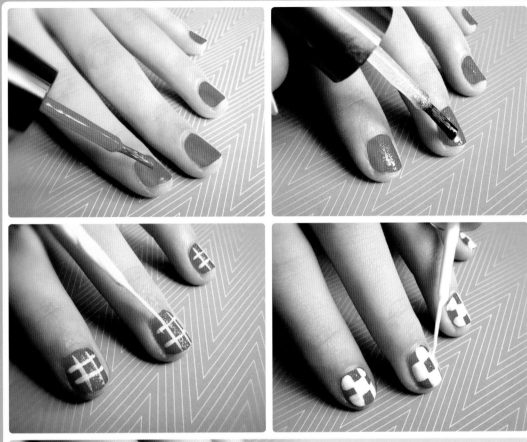

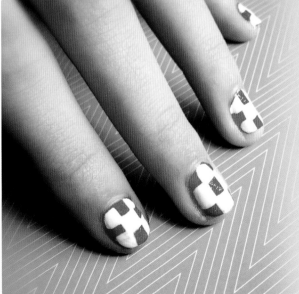

Pair two complimentary
colors for harmonious
balance. Try orange
with aqua and violet
with yellow.

argyle

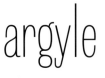

This classic print has been gracing sweaters worldwide for centuries. Yes, its preppy and just a little posh, but on your fingernails it becomes instantly edgy and cool. Try it and see for yourself!

TOOLS

Base coat

Color polish

Top coat

Water-based acrylic paint in three colors

Pencil

Angled brush

Striper brush

1) Apply base coat and two coats of color polish. Let dry.

2) Using your angled brush and acrylic paint, create two to three diamonds in a vertical row. (Whether you use two or three will depend on the size of your nail.)

3) Find the middle of each diamond and mark it with a pencil. Put a small mark in the middle of each side of each diamond as well.

4) Using your striper brush and another acrylic paint color, paint diagonal lines across the diamonds, using the pencil marks as a guide. The lines should extend past the diamonds, creating "X" shapes across the nail.

5) Let paint dry completely and apply top coat.

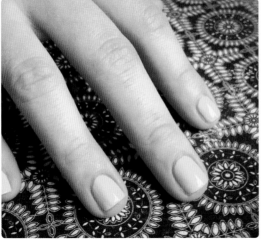

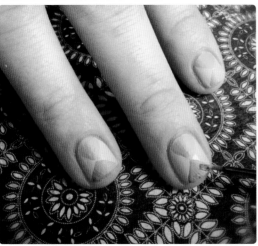

For this look, I'm using shades of yellow and blue. You can also try pink and mint green for that preppy-girl look, or dark red and blue for traditional scholarly style!

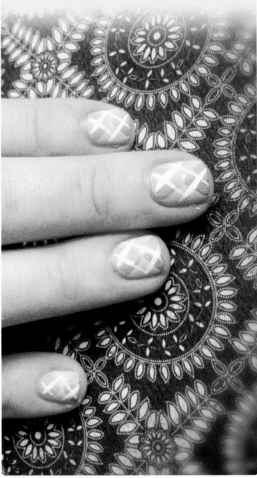

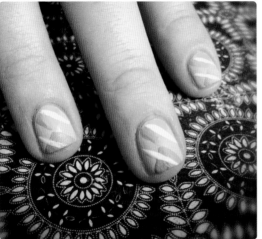

plaid

This traditional Scottish pattern is adored by all, be they preppy, Goth, urban, or hipster. Even with its private school ties and fifth-century beginnings, plaid will always have a slightly rebellious edge.

TOOLS

Base coat

Base polish color

Top coat

Four complementary shades of water-based acrylic paint

Wide nail art brush

Striper brush

1) Apply base coat and two coats of base polish color. Let polish dry.

2) Using your wide nail art brush and one color of acrylic paint, apply one thick stripe, vertically or horizontally, off-center.

3) Using your striper brush and the same color, apply two thin stripes in the opposite direction of the thick stripe. These two stripes should be close together, but not touching.

4) Using the same color, paint one thick stripe on the other side, and one crossing it in the opposite direction.

5) Clean your striper brush and, using another color, paint two more stripes: one between the first two, and one across it.

6) Let polish dry and apply top coat.

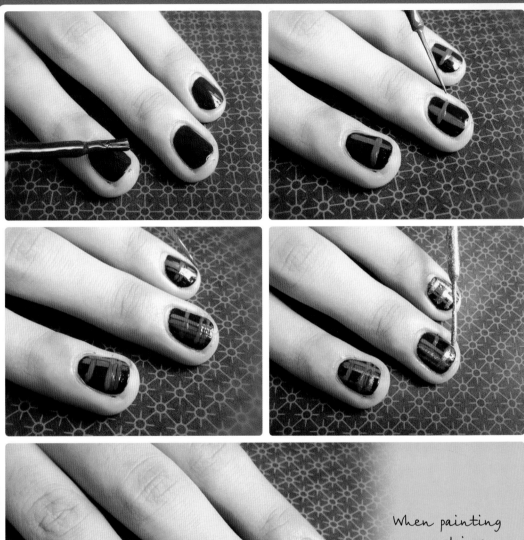

When painting
your stripes,
don't go over-
board. For the
best result,
keep it to six
stripes.

geometric shapes

As a lover of abstract art and a dedicated nonconform-ist, I have a particular fondness for the strong forms and clean lines of geometric shapes. They are quite striking when painted on your nails! Add colors and layering, and you've got all the ingredients you need to create some mind-blowing nail art.

TOOLS

Base coat

Base polish color (optional)

Nail art polish in your choice of several colors

Top coat

1) Apply base coat and two coats of base color polish, if desired. (I prefer clear nails with this design!) Let base coat and color dry completely. Unscrew the tops of the nail art polish bottles for easier access.

2) Paint a randomly placed triangle on each nail. Let dry.

3) Using another color, paint another triangle on each nail and let dry. Continue covering each nail with a series of different-colored triangles. You can bor-der some nails with triangles, cover the nail plate in overlapping triangles, or paint the triangles edge to edge like a pinwheel. Make every nail different! Let polish dry between each application.

4) Apply top coat and let dry.

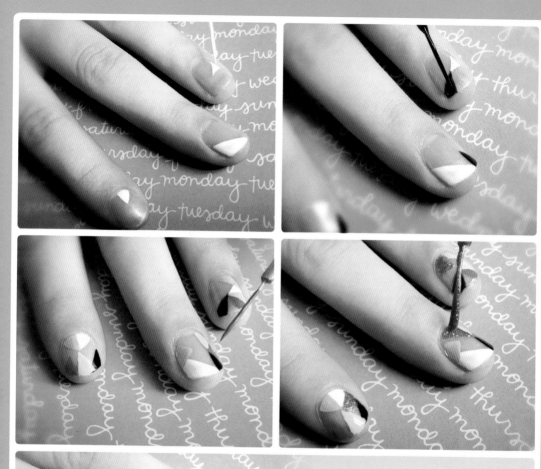

To keep this design from looking too busy, stick to three or four colors. Paint one triangle in a metallic or glitter color to really make the design pop!

stars and stripes

What symbol is more patriotic then an American flag? It's an icon and a fashion statement worn all over the world. According to legend, the red symbolizes valor, the white represents purity, and the blue stands for vigilance, perseverance, and justice. Who wouldn't want to embody those values on their nails?

TOOLS

Base coat

White polish

Top coat

Water-based acrylic paint in red, white, and blue

Striper brush

Thick flat brush

Dotter or toothpick

1) Apply base coat and two coats of white polish. Let dry.

2) Using a striper brush and red water-based acrylic paint, slowly glide on vertical stripes. Space them evenly apart so the lines between become the white stripes.

3) Using a thick flat brush and blue paint or polish, carefully paint a square across the free edge.

4) Using a dotter or toothpick and white paint, add white dots to the blue square, representing stars.

5) Let dry and apply top coat.

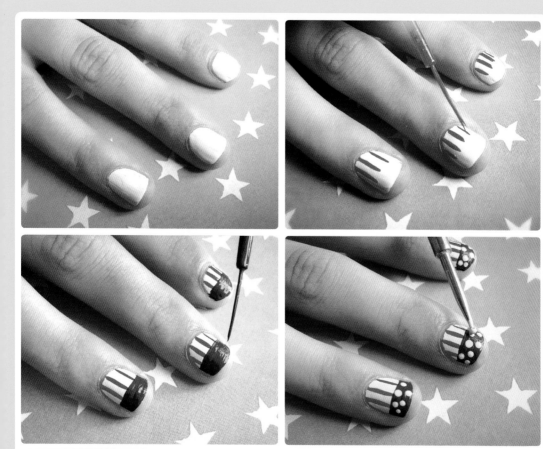

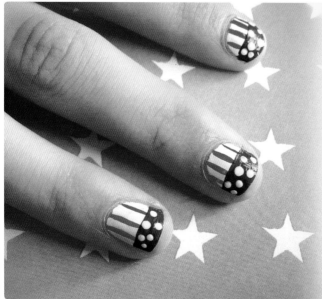

Experiment with
nail art inspired
by international
flags! Show pride
in your country
of origin, or pay
homage to a
favorite travel
destination.

tribal

Tribal prints are a key source of inspiration for fashion designers. They express style, fashion, and beauty across cultures and time. Take this stylish print off the rack and apply it to your fingertips!

TOOLS

Base coat

Color polish

Nail art polish in three to five colors

Top coat

1) Apply base coat and let dry.

2) Paint a geometric shape on each nail. Try a stripe, crescent, triangle, or semi-circle.

3) Use another polish color to outline one edge of each shape.

4) Using a third polish color, add tiny dots and dashes along another edge of each shape.

5) Add additional details by creating more tiny dots and dashes. Get creative and vary the design on each nail.

6) Let dry and apply top coat.

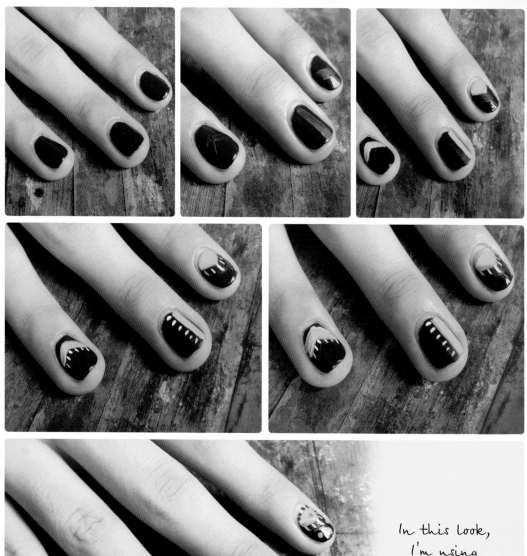

In this look,
I'm using
black polish
to make
my colorful
designs pop!

art deco

If you're looking for a glamorous, sexy design, and you long for the decadence of the Roaring '20s, then this Art Deco style is just up your alley!

TOOLS

Base coat

Base color polish

Black polish

Top coat

Gold studs

Striper brush

Tweezers

1) Apply base coat. Apply two coats of base color polish to all but the first nail on each hand. Paint these two nails black. Let dry.

2) Using a striper brush and black polish, paint diagonal lines across your third nail on each hand. Paint diagonal lines in the opposite direction. Let dry.

3) Apply a heavy coat of top coat on your first and third nails.

4) While the top coat is still wet and sticky, use tweezers to apply gold studs to the points on the third nail where the lines cross.

5) Use tweezers to apply gold studs across the painted black nail.

6) Press the studs into place using the tweezers.

7) Apply top coat over all nails and let dry.

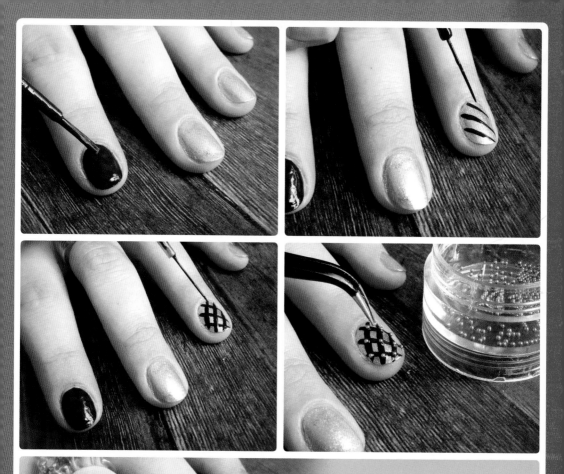

Instead of tweezers, try using a wooden pusher dipped in a little clear topcoat to make the studs easier to pick up.

rock star

Whether you're strumming a guitar or just typing on your computer, this design will surely remind you to rock on!

TOOLS

Base coat

Color polish

Top coat

Striper tape

Metal studs

Tweezers

1) Apply base coat and two coats of color polish.

2) Apply nail art striper tape in a "V" formation on each nail.

3) Apply top coat. While the polish is still tacky, use tweezers to apply three metal studs along the curve of cuticle, inside the "V". Apply one stud at the point of the "V".

4) Apply top coat and let dry.

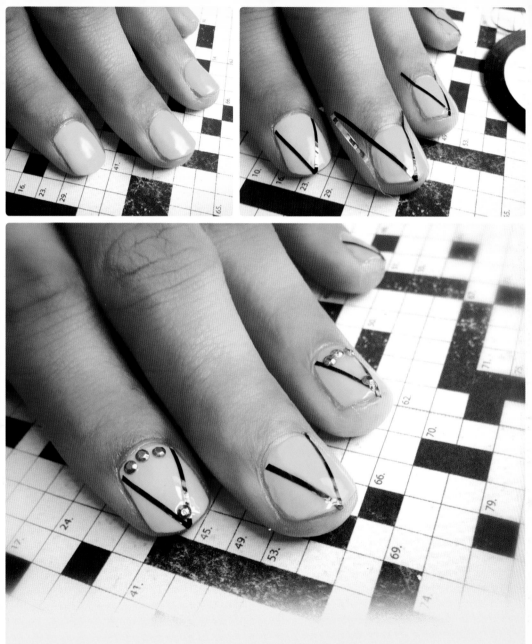

For this look, I used Illamasqua Nail Varnish in Rare.

nautical stripes

Nautical nails are a great look for spring and summer! They just scream beach vacation. Nautical stripes remind me of vacationing in the Hamptons, where stripes of blue, white, yellow, and red line the shores. Nautical stripes are trendy yet classic at the same time. By the time you pass this book down to your great-great-granddaughters, this look will still be in style!

TOOLS

Base coat

Color polish in white and blue

Top coat

Water-based acrylic paint in red and black

Detail brush

1) Apply base coat and let dry.

2) Using a detail brush, paint evenly spaced blue and white horizontal stripes.

3) Paint your ring fingernail white.

4) Use a detail brush to paint a small anchor anywhere on the nail. I like to use red water-based acrylic paint. An anchor is basically a lollypop with a "u" underneath. Add a black dot to the top of the anchor.

5) Let dry and apply top coat.

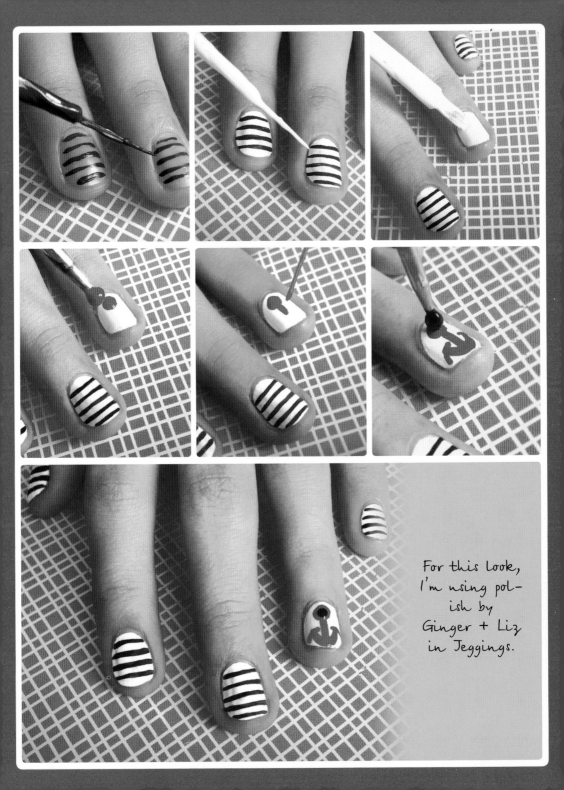

For this look,
I'm using pol-
ish by
Ginger + Liz
in Jeggings.

smiley face

A smiley face is an international symbol of happiness and goodwill. We use them most often in text messages and e-mail, but put them on your nails and I guarantee you won't need emoticons to express your cheer.

TOOLS

Base coat

Base color polish in bright yellow

Top coat

Water-based acrylic paint in black and red

Dotter or toothpick

Detail brush

1) Apply base coat and two coats of yellow base color polish. Let dry.

2) Dip a dotter or toothpick in black acrylic paint and create two long ovals close together for the eyes.

3) Using a detail brush, paint a large curved line under the two ovals. Add a small curved line on each side of the large one.

4) Using the dotter or toothpick, paint two tiny white dots on the tips of the ovals to create pupils. Add a tongue for a burst of silliness! Outline it in black to make it pop.

5) Let dry and apply top coat.

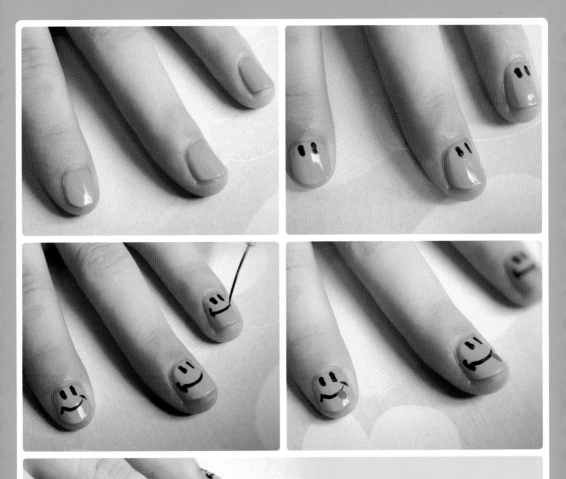

For a bright cheery
yellow, I'm using
Ginger + Liz
polish in Caution.

paris is for lovers

Pay homage to Paris, the city of love, and paint hearts on the tips of your French manicure. Top it off with some polka dots and shimmery accents for true Parisian flair.

TOOLS

Base coat

Base color polish in neutral shade

Color polish in two to six shades

Glitter nail art polish

Dotter or toothpick

1) Apply base coat and one coat of neutral base color polish.

2) Paint two curved lines on the free edge of the nail plate. To do this, hold the brush vertically on one side of the side wall and sweep the brush down and in toward the middle. Repeat on the other side. You should have a shape that resembles the top of a heart.

3) Using glitter nail art polish, outline the top of the heart.

4) Using a dotter or toothpick, apply dots to the empty space above the heart.

5) Let dry and apply top coat.

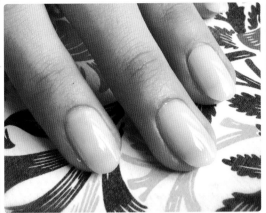

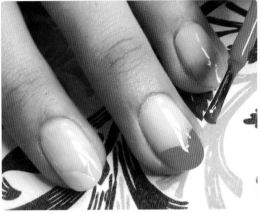

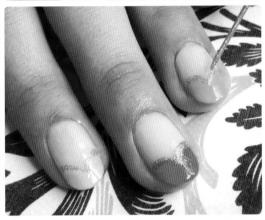

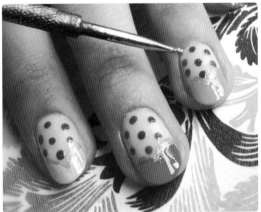

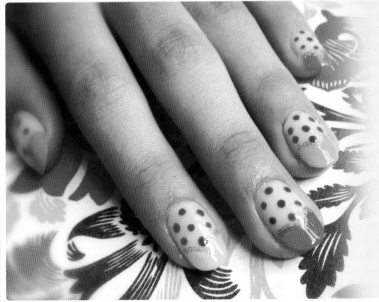

For this look, I went wild with a different look on each nail! You can also scale back the color scheme and use the same shade on each nail.

up in flames

Not all girls love pink, glitter, and ponies; some chicks prefer leather over lace. If you're that kind of gal, then this tutorial is for you. Flame on, rock star!

TOOLS

Base coat

Base color polish

Top coat

Water-based acrylic paint in red, orange, yellow, black, and burgundy

Small flat nail art brush

Detail brush

1) Apply base coat and two coats of black or dark-colored nail polish. (Dark colors will add intensity to the fire!)

2) We're going to make the free edge the starting point for the flame. Using your small flat brush and the lightest yellow color, paint "S" shapes from free edge to free edge, joining them together midway from the base to form one big flame.

3) Repeat step two with each additional color, starting with the lightest and ending with the deepest. Layer each color on top of the other with some of the previous color exposed.

4) Using a detail brush, paint the edges of the fire in black or burgundy. This gives the design shape and movement.

5) Let your design dry and apply top coat.

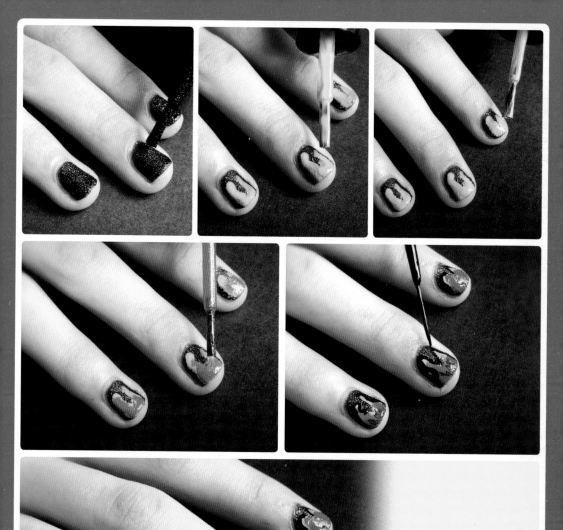

For this look,
I'm going
with a rockin'
black polish
to highlight the
fiery flames.

vintage lace

If vintage-chic is your style, look to lace for nail art inspiration. Study a piece of lace and you'll see how every shape shares a wall with the one next to it in order to create a gorgeous pattern.

TOOLS

Base coat

Base color polish

Water-based acrylic paint

Top coat

Striper brush

Dotter or toothpick

1) Apply base coat and two coats of base color polish. Let dry.

2) Using your striper brush and acrylic paint, paint two wavy lines with one to two peaks, from free edge to free edge, equally spaced apart.

3) Paint diagonal crossing lines below the lower wavy line, closest to the free edge.

4) Using a dotter or toothpick, create a line of dots across the upper wavy line.

5) Let dry and apply top coat.

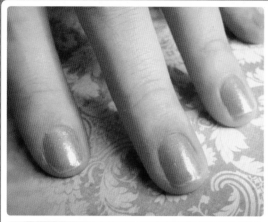

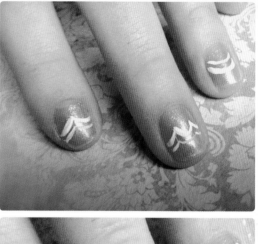

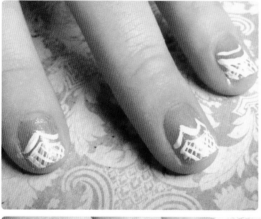

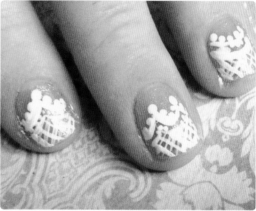

White lace evokes
free-spirited
innocence and
nostalgia for the
past. For a more
sexy, sultry look,
black lace is
every girl's secret
weapon.

frosted cupcake

How sweet is this design? All the delicious appeal of a real cupcake without the sugar rush? Sounds like a great treat to me!

TOOLS

Base coat

Color polish

Top coat

Water-based acrylic paint in colors of your choice

Angled brush

Detail brush

Large dotter

1) Apply base and two coats of color polish. Let dry.

2) Using an angled brush and acrylic paint, create one thick horizontal stripe across the bottom half of the nail, covering the free edge.

3) Using a color one shade lighter, paint on three to four vertical stripes over the acrylic paint.

4) Using large dotter, make a row of overlapping dots along the top edge of your design.

5) Using a detail brush and the same color of paint, create a curved line on top of your dots from free edge to free edge. Fill it in and let dry.

6) Using a toothpick, poke randomly scattered multi-colored dots on top of the frosting to resemble sprinkles.

7) Using your large dotter and red paint, add a cherry on top. Use the detail brush to draw a stem.

8) Let dry and apply top coat.

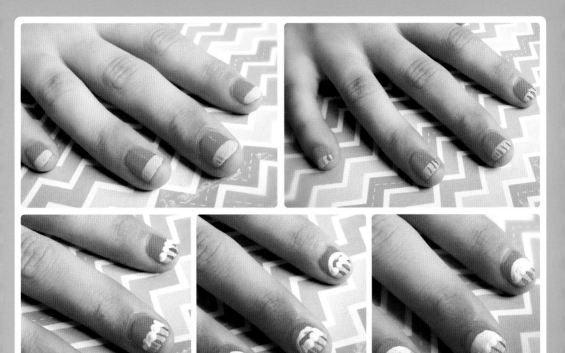

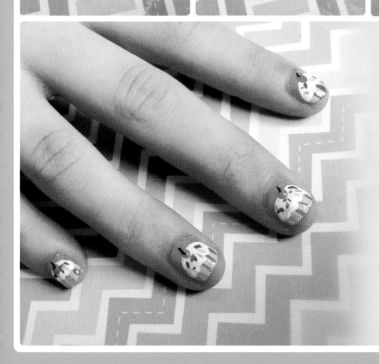

Here I'm using white paint to resemble vanilla icing, but you can try brown for chocolate, pink for strawberry, or any color you like.

puzzle

If you're looking for a playful design, this one is it! Don't be puzzled by its application, though; it's much easier to put together than the ones that come in a box.

TOOLS

Base coat

Top coat

Water-based acrylic paint in black, and four more colors of your choice

Detail brush

Medium and small dotter

Painter's tape

1) Apply a thin coat of base coat. Cut a small strip of painter's tape and place it horizontally across the bottom half of the nail plate. Choose two paint colors and paint one swipe of each, side by side, on the uncovered area of the nail, then remove the tape.

2) On the bottom bare half of your nail, carefully paint on the other two colors in the same style as the previous step.

3) Using a detail brush and black paint, paint the borders (the lines where the blocks of color meet). Now you should have a cross in the middle of your nails.

4) Using a dotter, add a black dot to the middle of each line. Let dry.

5) Using a small dotter or tooth pick, paint each black dot the same color as the square next to it, but don't cover it completely; leave a border that creates the round part where the puzzle pieces join.

6) Let dry and apply top coat.

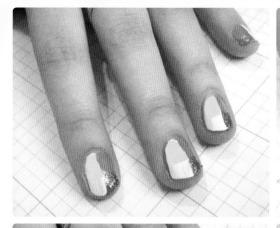

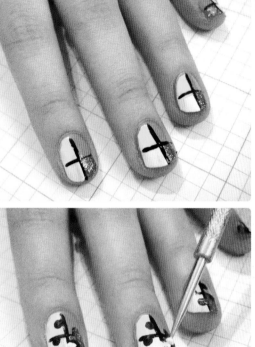

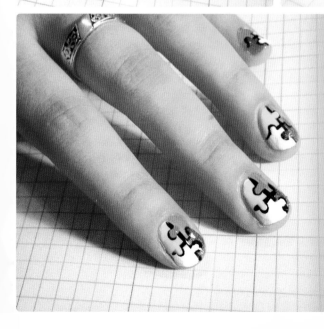

Puzzled by which four colors to use? Refer to your color wheel! Use white or black and then pick three analogous colors (three colors that sit side by side, like green, blue, and purple).

springtime flowers

Enjoy the vibrancy and liveliness of spring, and don't worry for a minute about allergies and itchy noses!

TOOLS

Base coat

Color polish in red and shimmery neutral

Nail art polish in red, pink, and green

Top coat

Water-based acrylic paint

1) Apply base coat and two coats of base polish color, alternating colors. Let polish dry.

2) Using red nail art polish, paint small clusters of semi-circles on the neutral nails.

3) Use pink nail art polish to add highlights.

4) Using green nail art polish, create one to two leaves around each flower by quickly flicking the brush out from the flower in short strokes.

5) Apply top coat and let dry.

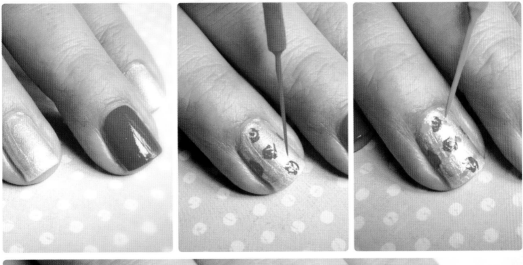

Pastel shades are an obvious choice when it comes to flowers and springtime. I like to shake things up, so in this look, I paired red with a shimmery neutral for an unexpectedly original color combination. Experiment with color to find your own striking color scheme.

summer fun

When I think of summer, I think of hot nights, trips to the fair, and ice cream trucks. Here I'm using colors and shapes to create the look and feel of a hot summer night.

TOOLS

Base coat

Water-based acrylic paint in red, blue, green, orange, purple, yellow, and white

Striper brush

Dotter or toothpick

Top coat

1) Apply base coat. Using the striper brush, paint long vertical red and white stripes from free edge to free edge.

2) Next break out your dotting tool and create little multicolored balls up and down one side of the nail. Make sure you use only one color at a time, and try not to go overboard with the amount of dots.

3) Lastly, dot a small cluster of balls on the free edge, creating a cascade formation.

4) Let dry and apply top coat.

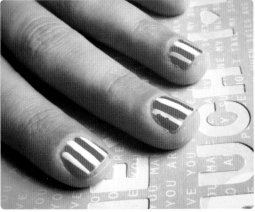
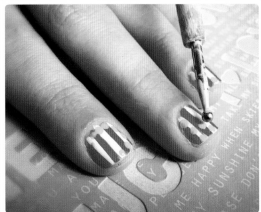
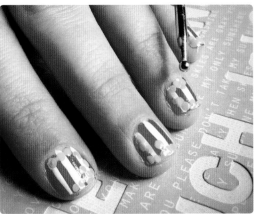
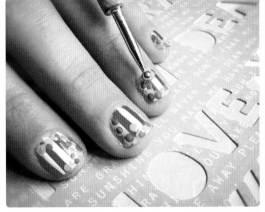
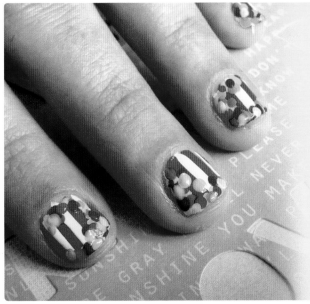

Take inspiration
from a carnival, and
go wild with color!

autumn leaves

Autumn is my favorite month of the year! The air gets crisp, school is back in session, and we get to break out our stylish coats—with stylish nails to match!

TOOLS

Base coat

Base polish color

Top coat

Nail art polish in red, orange, yellow, and gold

1) Apply base coat and two coats of color polish, but keep one accent nail clear.

2) On your accent nail, use yellow nail art polish to paint three to four pointed oval shapes scattered across the nail. Let polish dry slightly.

3) Repeat step two with each color, leaving a bit of drying time between each color.

4) Create a thin line down the middle of some leaves to add detail.

5) Apply top coat and let dry.

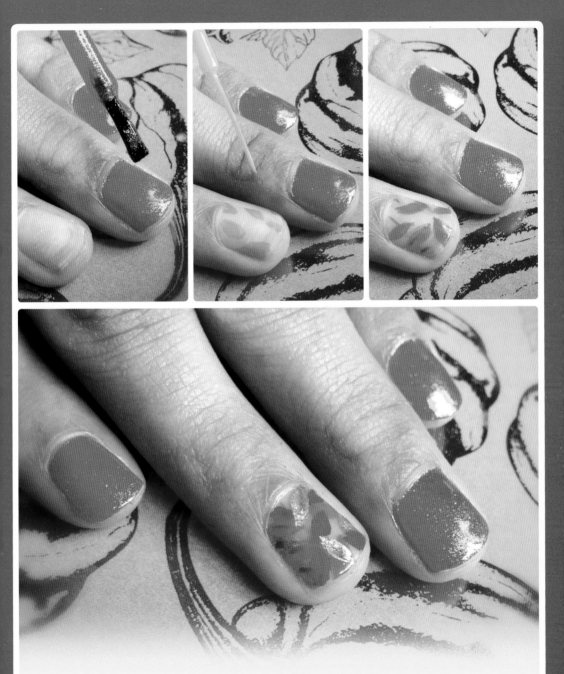

The colors of this season are deep, rich, and warm.
As a base color, here I'm using "Amy" by Zoya.

let it snow

Polish away those winter blues with sparkle and snow-flakes. Although winter can be cold and harsh, this design captures the beauty of freshly fallen snow.

TOOLS

Base coat

Base polish color

White nail art polish

Top coat

Dotter or toothpick

1) Apply base coat and two coats of color polish. Let polish dry.

2) Using white nail art polish, paint "X" shapes on each nail. Create variety by painting them in different sizes and locations on the nail.

3) Paint two tiny "V" shapes along the lines of the "X", with points toward the center of each "X".

4) Using a dotter or toothpick, scatter white dots around the snowflakes.

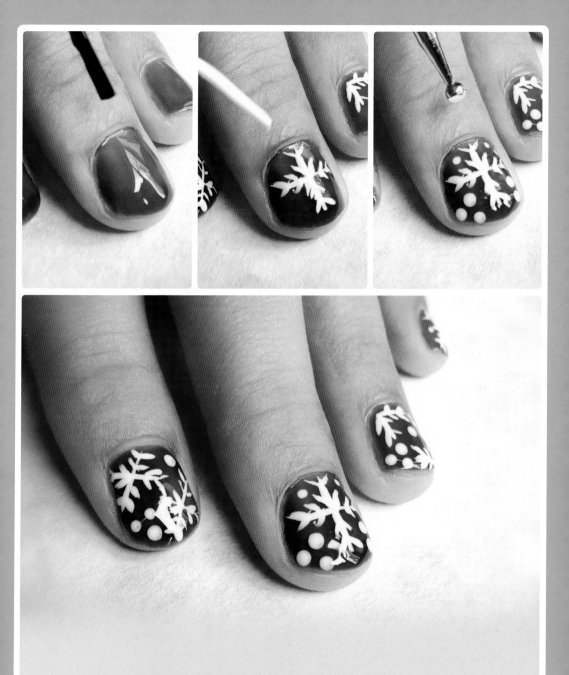

For a whimsical winter look, I used a blue-green color
called Frida by Zoya.

pow!

Transform your nails into a knockout statement piece! This design lets everyone know you are a force to be reckoned with.

TOOLS

Base coat

Glitter polish

Black nail art polish

Water-based acrylic paint in white and yellow

Flat nail art brush

Makeup wedge sponge

1) Apply base coat and two coats of glitter polish. Let dry.

2) Using a flat nail art brush and white acrylic paint, create a partial star in the lower right corner of the middle fingernail and the lower left corner of the ring fingernail.

3) Using a makeup wedge sponge, apply yellow paint to the center of the star.

4) Using black nail art polish, outline the yellow paint with open triangles.

5) Using black nail art polish, write "POW" on the middle nail. Paint an exclamation point on the other the nail. Let dry.

6) Apply top coat and let dry.

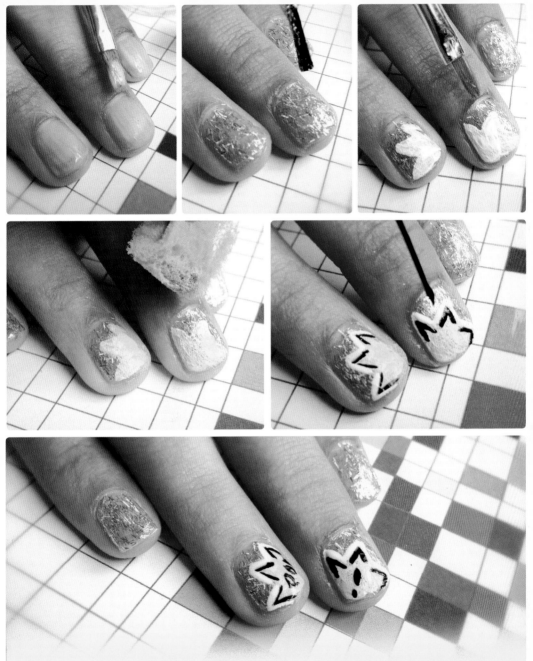

Try using Illamasqua Nail Varnish in Harsh, and you'll really knock everyone out!

beauty queen

So maybe you can't wear your real crown in public. This nail design is a great way to add a royal touch to your look, while still keeping it subtle.

TOOLS

Base coat

Base color polish

Water-based acrylic paint in white, yellow, pink, and gray

Top coat

Detail brush

Dotter or toothpick

1) Apply base coat and two coats of base color polish. Let dry.

2) Using a detail brush, paint a curved line from free edge to free edge about one third of the way up. This will be the base of your crown.

3) In the center of the curve, paint a straight vertical line stopping just before the cuticle. This will be the highest point of the crown.

4) Using the middle line as a guide, paint a tall center triangle.

5) To the left of the center triangle, paint two small overlapping triangles. Repeat with two more small overlapping triangles on the right. Fill in the centers.

6) Using your dotting tool, make a dot on the tip of each point.

7) Using a detail brush, outline your whole design.

8) Let dry and apply top coat.

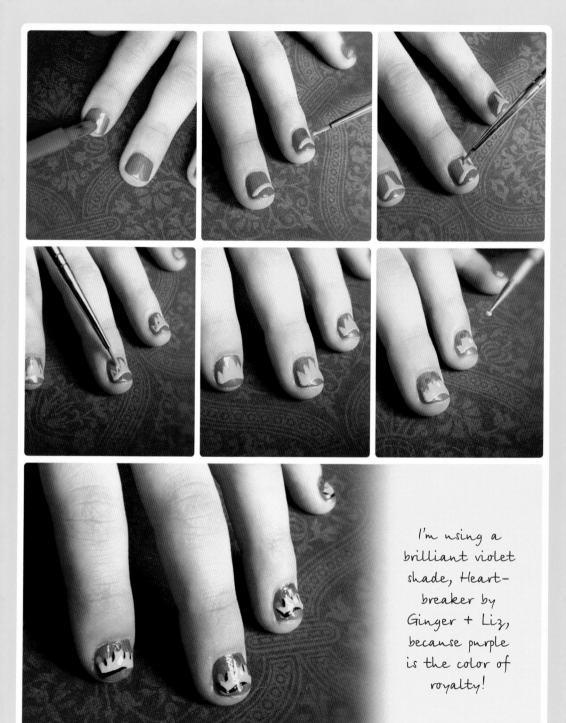

I'm using a brilliant violet shade, Heart-breaker by Ginger + Liz, because purple is the color of royalty!

pucker up

Nothing says glam like perfect red puckers. They truly never go out of style. But if you're not bold enough (or old enough) to rock the red lip look on your face, why not give it a test run on your nails?

TOOLS

Base coat

Polish color

Top coat

Water-based acrylic paint in red, white, and black

Detail brush

Pencil

1) Apply base coat and two coats of base color polish. Let dry.

2) Choose a location on the nail plate for your design. Using a detail brush, slowly paint a curved line for the bottom lip.

3) Paint a curved line with two humps for the upper lip. Let dry.

4) After your color dries, grab a pencil and sketch out your details. You can create as many or as few details as you like. Keep in mind, natural lips have grooves and creases.

5) Using a detail brush and white paint, add highlights where the light would hit the curve of the lips.

6) Using a detail brush, go over your pencil marks with black paint.

7) Let dry completely and apply top coat.

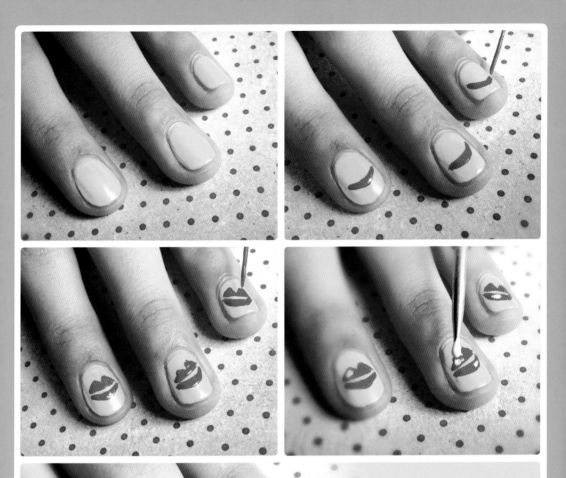

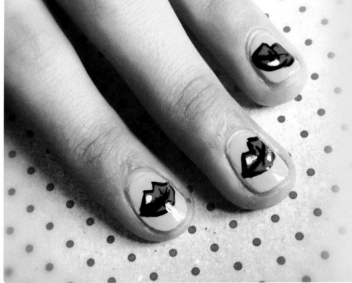

To highlight these look-at-me lips, I'm going with a show-stopping neon yellow base color, Never a Dull Moment by Ginger + Liz.

tootie fruity

Fruit is beautiful in its own right, but when painted on your nails, it's yummy to look at, and stylish to boot!

TOOLS

Base coat

Base polish color in a neutral shade

Top coat

Water-based acrylic paint in shades of orange, red, and green

White nail art polish

Nail art brush

Detail brush

Pencil

1) Apply base coat and one coat of base color. Let polish dry.

2) Using water-based acrylic paint and a nail art brush, create an orange semi-circle, a red triangle, and a green circle, overlapping the shapes to create dimension. Let dry.

3) Using a pencil, sketch in the details of the fruit.

4) Using a detail brush, fill in your sketches with lighter complementary shades.

5) Add more detail with thin outlines.

6) Let dry and apply top coat.

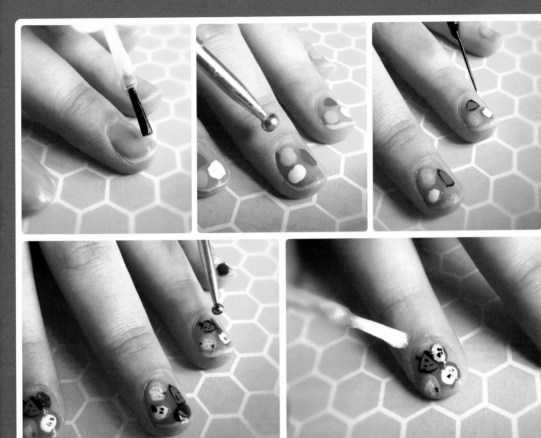

The fruit is the focus of this design, so I'm keeping the background simple with a neutral shade.

crystal flowers

With this gorgeous, sparkly design, you can enjoy a dazzling field of flowers any time of year.

TOOLS

Base coat

Color polish

Nail art polish in light and dark green

Top coat

Rhinestones in a variety of colors and shapes

Wooden pusher

Tweezers

1) Apply base coat and two coats of color polish.

2) Using light and dark green nail art polish, flick vertical stripes from the free edge, one-third of the way up the nail plate. Don't try to be too precise, because you're creating natural flower stems and grass. Let dry and apply a heavy layer of top coat.

3) While the top coat is still wet, use tweezers to pick up and place multicolored rhinestones atop the stems.

4) Using a wooden pusher, secure the stones by gently pressing them into place.

5) Apply top coat around the stones and over the painted portion of the nail plate. Painting over the stones will dull their glimmer.

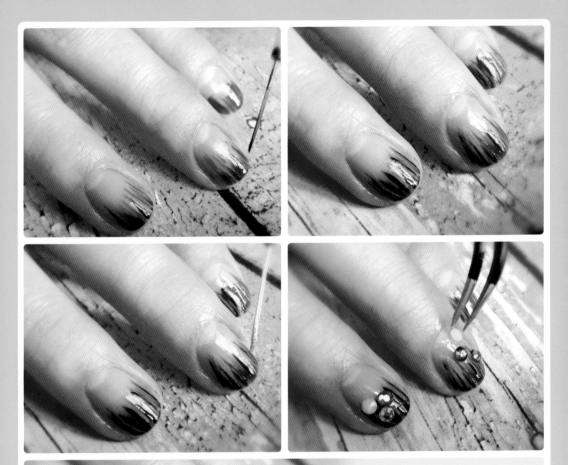

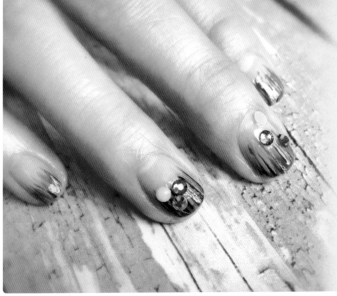

With a complex, blinged-out design like this, I prefer to decorate just two or three nails. But use your creativity and feel free to go wild!

court jester

No clowning around with this design! It's fully festive and totally easy. Don't worry if your painting skills are not up to par, just let the tape do all the work for you.

TOOLS

Base coat

Metallic gold color polish

Top coat

Nail striper tape

Acrylic paint in pink and purple

Makeup wedge sponge

Gold studs

Tweezers

1) Apply base coat. Apply two coats of metallic polish to every other nail.

2) On the remaining nails, use nail striper tape and place it in a diagonal crisscross pattern.

3) Using a makeup wedge sponge and pink acrylic paint, sponge paint over the taped nails. Repeat with purple acrylic paint. Slowly remove tape.

4) Apply top coat to the nails with the tape designs. While the top coat is still wet, use tweezers to apply studs at the points where the lines intersect.

5) Apply top coat to the remaining nails and let dry.

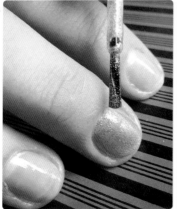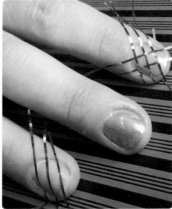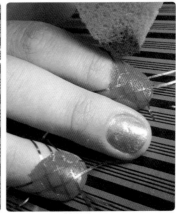
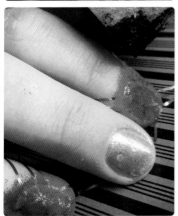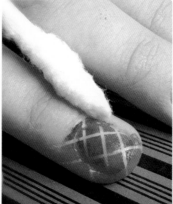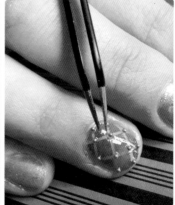

For this look, I'm using Illamasqua Nail Varnish in Spartan.

dark crystal

If you love adorning your ears, neck, and wrists with dark and dramatic jewels, then darling, you must try it on your tips.

TOOLS

Base coat

Color polish in a sparkly black hue

Top coat

Assorted gems, crystals, and studs

Tweezers

1) Apply base coat and two coats of color polish.

2) Apply top coat. While the top coat is still wet, use tweezers to place gems and crystals in various jewel-like patterns on your first and ring fingernails. I recommend you start by placing the largest stones.

3) Next, place the smallest stones around the larger ones. Lastly, use additional stones as accents.

4) Using tweezers, gently press the stones into the wet polish to secure them in place. Let dry.

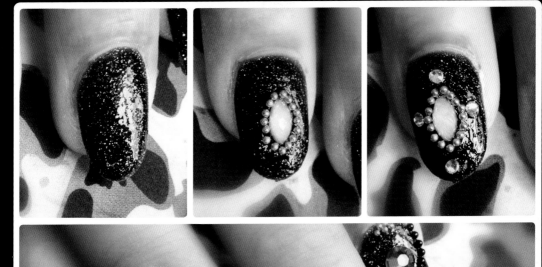

Take inspiration from jewelry to create this look. Emulate
Audrey Hepburn from *Breakfast at Tiffany's* as you browse the
display cases of fine jewelry stores, croissant in hand. Then
create an affordable version at home on your nails!

Choose metal studs that complement your jewelry.
If you typically wear yellow gold, then choose studs to match.
If you're rocking silver, platinum, or white gold, use studs
with a similar finish.

modern pop

Bring on the British Invasion! Lets play homage to the Mods of the Swinging '60s with this jive nail design.

TOOLS

Base coat

Color polish in two shades

Nail art polish in black, gold, and another complementary color

Top coat

1) Apply base coat. Paint six fingers with one color of polish, and the remaining four with the other color.

2) Next, grab two of your nail art polish colors and pair them up with the shades of color polish already painted on your nails. I'm pairing pink with gold and green with lavender.

3) Paint small crescent shapes right above each cuticle, covering about one-fourth of the nail plate.

4) Using black nail art polish, outline the perimeters of each nail and the crescents.

5) Let dry and apply top coat.

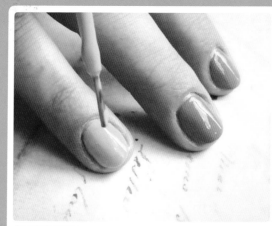

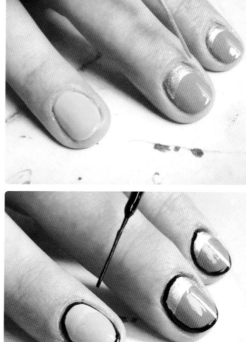

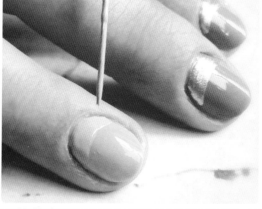

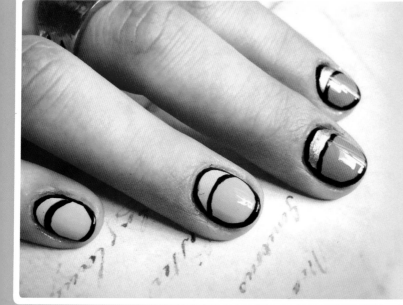

For this look, I'm using bright pastel hues, like American Apparel nail polish in Office and Rose Bowl.

retro cartoon

Roy Lichtenstein brought comic strips and cartoons to the art world with the Pop Art movement. Let's bring that look to our nails with a design that any Betty or Veronica would covet.

TOOLS

Base coat

Color polish in red

Nail art polish in black and white

Top coat

Dotter or toothpick

1) Apply base coat and two coats of color polish.

2) Outline the perimeter of each nail in black.

3) Using a dotter or toothpick, paint a white dot in the same corner on each nail.

4) Using white nail art polish, paint a highlight extending from the dot on each nail.

5) Let dry and apply top coat.

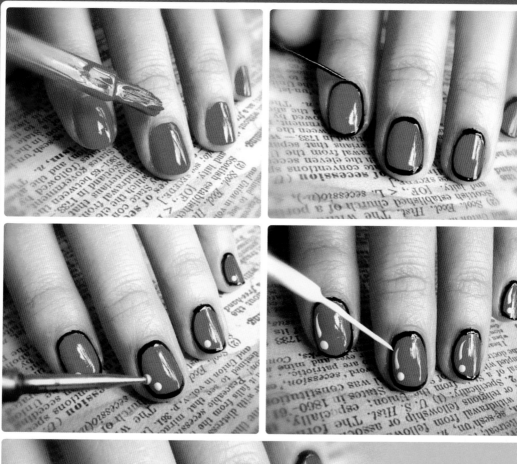

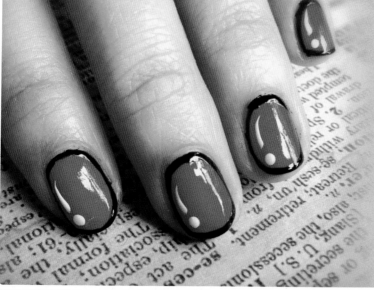

For a perfectly smooth, even coat of color polish, always start painting in the middle of your nail plate. This will give the polish on the brush room to spread.

haute couture

When you hear the word "couture," you know something chic is about to follow. These "haute" nails take chic to a whole new level.

TOOLS

Base coat

Color polish

Top coat

Nail decals

Nail chain

Flat back pearls

Nail glue

Tweezers

1) Cut out two nail decals. Measure and cut four pieces of nail chain to create an arc across the width of your nail plate.

2) Apply base coat and two coats of color polish.

3) While the polish is still wet, slowly apply the decal to the middle nail.

4) Apply top coat. Immediately place a piece of nail chain on the nail plate of the first and ring fingers, in an arc to form a necklace. Press it into place.

5) Add a small dot of nail glue above and below the nail chain. Using tweezers, apply pearls and press gently to adhere them to the glue.

6) Apply another coat of top coat and let dry.

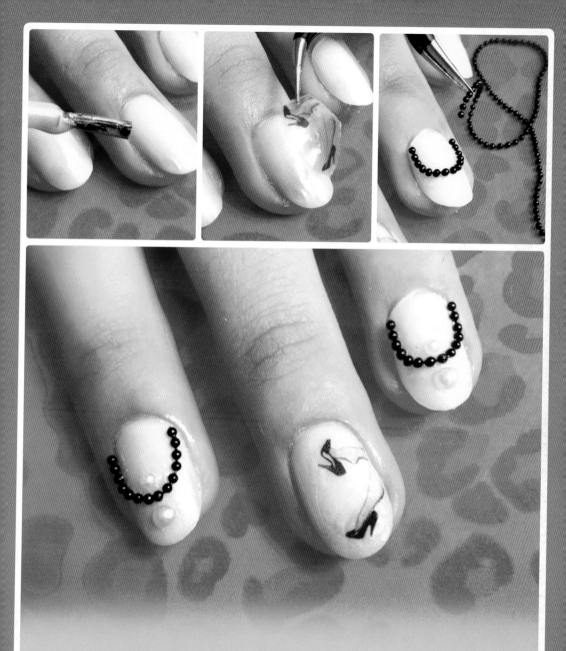

For this look, I'm using Illamasqua Nail Varnish
in Monogamous.

gilded city

Gold symbolizes wealth, glitz, and outstanding merit. As a kid, getting a gold star makes you feel outstanding, and these glitzy nails have the same effect.

TOOLS

Base coat

Gold metallic polish

Gold glitter top coat

Black nail art polish

Top coat

Crystals

Metal studs

Tweezers

1) Lay out your crystals and studs in the pattern you want to create. Use the image to the right, or create your own design.

2) Apply base coat and two coats of gold metallic polish.

3) Apply glitter top coat. Let dry.

4) Using black nail art polish, paint a thin horizontal line across each nail, one-fourth of the way back from the free edge. Skip the ring fingernail, as this will be your accent nail.

5) Apply clear top coat to all nails.

6) While the polish is still wet, use tweezers to apply crystals and studs to the accent nail. Start from the center and work your way out, completely filling the nail plate with your embellishments.

7) Gently press them into place using tweezers. Let dry.

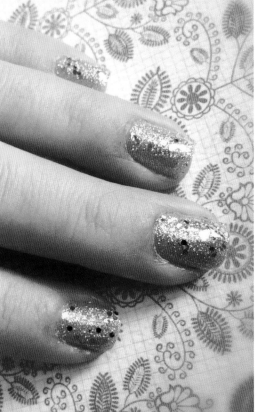

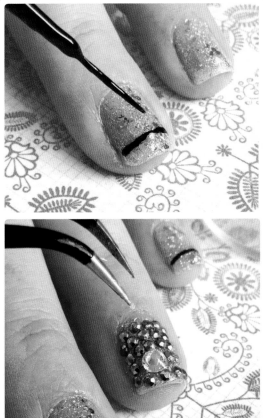

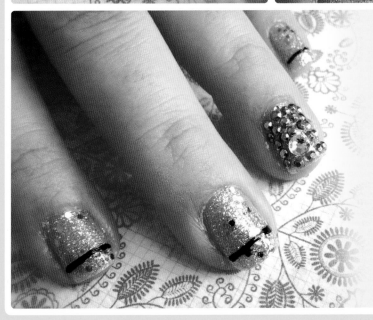

For this look, I used Zoya Nail Polish in Kerry for the metallic polish, and Sephora by OPI glitter top coat in Only Gold for Me.

✗ FINDING INSPIRATION

After seeing all this slamming nail art, you may be wondering how you're going to come up with equally creative designs on your own. Well, let me tell you, inspiration doesn't just fall into an artist's lap; a true nail artist must get out there and find it! Nail art clearly isn't a new idea; millions of incredible designs are available in magazines, on billboards, and all over the internet. But there are hundreds, nay, *thousands* of dazzling nail art concepts just waiting to be discovered! To create an extraordinary design, your best bet is to look in unusual places. Here are ten noteworthy ideas to help get you started on your quest to find some truly stellar and unique nail art inspiration.

→ ## Greeting Cards

The prime purpose of greeting cards is to express messages with images, using just a few words, if any. Like nail art, they are usually themed-based and full of colorful, creative, and cute designs.

→ ## Gift-wrapping Paper

Like greeting cards, gift-wrapping paper is covered with images following a particular theme, designed to convey excitement and curiosity. Wrapping paper is an excellent source for holiday and birthday inspiration.

→ ## Past Eras

Imagine America in the 1920s; what comes to mind? For me, it's *The Great Gatsby*, Art Deco style, beads, pearls, and champagne. Now consider the 1980s: neon, cassette tapes, and Valley girls. Each era has a unique style with particular motifs that are great for design ideas.

→ ## Nature

You don't need me to tell you that nature is the ultimate source for design inspiration. I'm talking about more than just the basic trees, flowers, and leaves. Nature can spark different ideas for texture, color, shape, and variation.

→ ## Children's Book Illustrations

Children's books are visually delicious, filled with vibrant colors and expressive styles to grab hold of easily distracted young minds. Take some time to revisit a few of your childhood faves. You'll get a surge of inspiration from the designs, and perhaps from the childhood memories too!

→ Fashion

Fashion is my favorite source of inspiration because it is always evolving; every season, designers set a new curve for what's cool. No matter what your style is, there's an exciting new look out there for you. Next time you flip through your favorite fashion mag, pay attention to the patterns, accessories, and current color schemes. These elements will help you create nail art designs to please the trendiest fashionista.

→ Album Covers

Album covers offer a variety of creative styles for design inspiration. They represent eras in time, portray emotion, and display style all at the same time. Your favorite music is an important part of your identity, so the art from your favorite albums is a perfect source for styling your own nails.

→ Architecture

If you're lucky to have spent time in an interesting city, I'm sure you've seen your share of cool buildings. Next time you're out and about, study the textures, shapes, colors, and lines of the world around you. No two structures are exactly the same. Draw inspiration from their odd shapes, unique colors, and historic features.

→ The Mall

Everything that can be sold is created with a particular design: clothing, jewelry, toys, and even food. Step into a clothing store and notice the shapes and patterns. Check out a toy store and notice colors, shapes, and themes. Even an everyday food market is full of interesting shapes and colors designed to make the food look delectable.

→ Yourself

Take a minute to look around your room. Appreciate the colors, the art on your walls, and the clothes in your closet. It's all you, baby! Your individuality and personal taste can be expressed in a million different ways with the flick of a lacquer brush. Think of your favorite flower, your school mascot, the friendship bracelet your best friend made; they all translate perfectly to nail design. Use your nails as a gallery to showcase your world!

more DIY inspiration

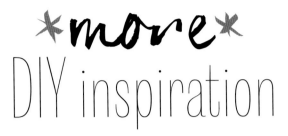

from RACE POINT PUBLISHING

Awesome nail art is everywhere these days! Check out street style snaps and online fashion blogs for the freshest ideas. DIY nail art aficionados are building their skills to rival the professionals, and with the tips in this book, you can too. Check out these amazing designs created at home and submitted in a contest hosted by Race Point Publishing via Instagram. Of all the incredible designs submitted, these 20 designs highlight the creativity, variety, and personal style that makes nail art so fabulous.

(1) yellowronni6	(6) yellowronni6	(11) little_haven	(16) honeybee_nails
(2) honeybee_nails	(7) little_haven	(12) little_haven	(17) jazzyliciouz_nailz
(3) yellowronni6	(8) planet_nikki	(13) little_haven	(18) glittermyfingers
(4) _skinnyy_mini	(9) little_haven	(14) katylouiseb_nails	(19) brie1284
(5) @katylouiseb	(10) yummycupcakes86	(15) honeybee_nails	(20) @michiesnails

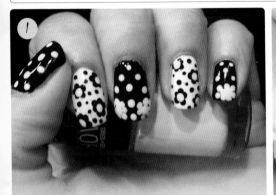

A floral design gets a tomboy-like update in royal blue.

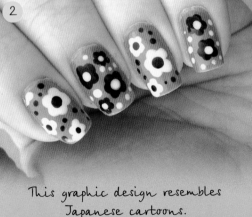

This graphic design resembles Japanese cartoons.

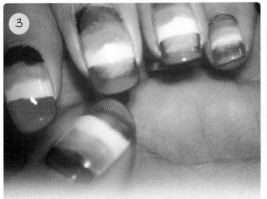

3

This look amps up an ombré design with a rainbow of shades.

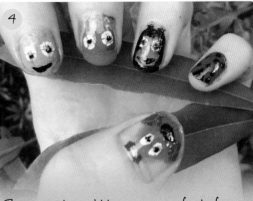

4

These cute critters are perfect for a child's manicure.

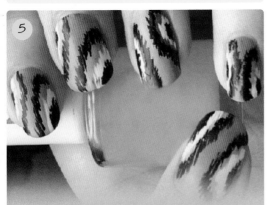

5

An ikat pattern is classic, modern, and perfectly on trend.

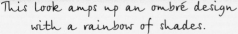

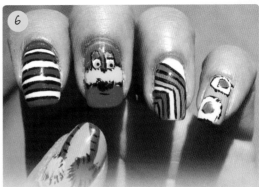

6

Pay homage to a favorite children's book, The Lorax, by Dr. Seuss.

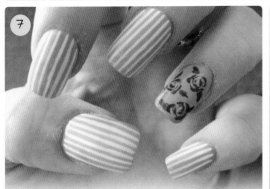

7

This preppy design calls for a mint julep on a sunny porch.

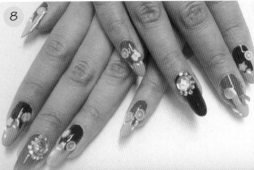

8

No such thing as too much bling? This design is for you!

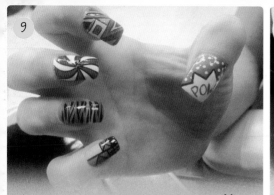

9

Showcase your skills with a different complex design on each nail.

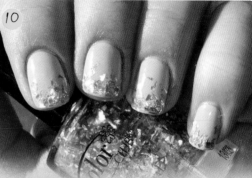

10

These cascading glitter tips are like shimmery winter icicles.

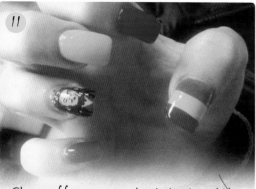

11

Show off your musical taste with a reggae tribute to Bob Marley.

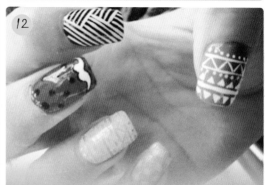

12

Take tribal print to a new level by varying the designs and color schemes.

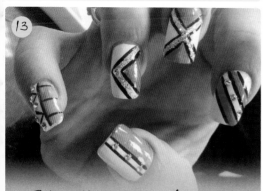

13

This striking design features graphic stripes, glitter, and studs.

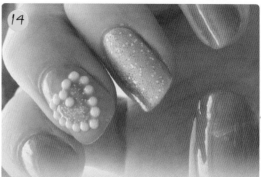

14

Pastels, hearts, and pearls say you're as sweet as can be.

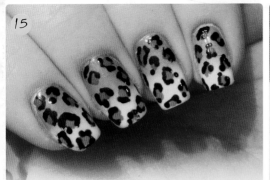

15

This daring look combines leopard spots with ombré in a strikingly offbeat color scheme.

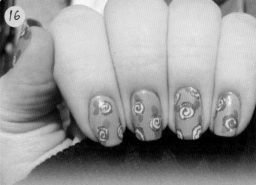

16

This look screams "granny-chic" with periwinkle and pink roses.

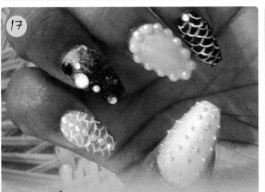

17

Give feminine pearls a masculine edge by pairing them with cobalt blue.

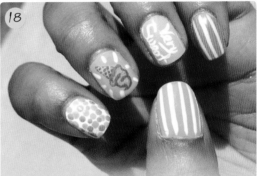

18

Take inspiration from a good old-fashioned ice cream parlor.

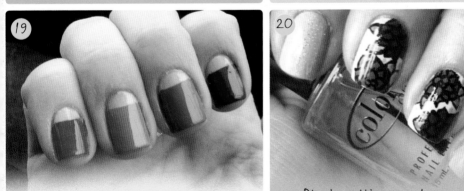

19

Glossy rainbow hues modernize the retro moon manicure.

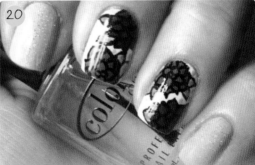

20

Black outlines and unexpected placement make this floral design graphic and edgy.

glossary

ACETONE: A colorless, flammable, liquid solvent that is an active ingredient in nail polish remover.

ARTIFICIAL TIPS: Coverings placed over natural nails to extend length. Used as a foundation for wraps, gel, and acrylic.

AROMATHERAPY: The practice of using scents to stimulate the brain and body. Aromatherapy is used to relieve a host of physical and emotional conditions, including stress, pain, insomnia, low energy, and infection.

BASE COAT: A coating that holds the nail polish onto the nail bed and prevents the polish from staining the nails.

BOTANICALS: Beneficial ingredients derived from nature.

BUFFER: Tool used to smooth the nail plate to create a more even and shiny surface.

CALLUS: Hard, thickened area of skin, usually resulting from friction.

CALLUS SOFTENER: Liquid gel that smooths rough spots on feet. Common active ingredients include lactic acid and sodium hydroxide.

CLIPPERS: Metal tool used for cutting fingernails and toenails.

CUTICLE: Semi-transparent dead tissues attached to the base of the nail plate.

CUTICLE REMOVER: Liquid or cream used to dissolve or loosen excess tissue from the nail plate, generally made up of 5 percent gentle acids.

FILE: Tool used to gently grind down and shape the edges of nails. Nail files can be emery boards, ceramic, glass, crystal, or metal.

FREE EDGE: The portion of the nail plate that extends past the nail bed.

FRENCH MANICURE: Manicure designed to resemble natural nails, with natural pink base nails and white tips.

GROWTH TREATMENT: Liquid polish treatment designed to support quicker natural nail growth, made with active ingredients proven to nourish the nail and nail bed.

HYPONYCHIUM: The seal located under the free edge that forms the curved line that shows through the nail plate.

INGROWN NAIL: Painful condition in which the nail grows into the nail bed, usually due to improper trimming of the nail by filling or cutting the nail too deep in the corners.

LUNULA: The half-moon shape located at the bottom of the nail near the cuticle.

MANICURE: Treatment to care for the hands and fingernails, including soaking, moisturizing, trimming, filing, and polishing.

MATRIX: The place at the base of the nail where nail growth originates and new nail cells are formed.

NAIL BED: The area beneath the nail plate composed of living tissues, blood vessels, and nerves.

NAIL GLUE: A bonder to fix cracks and adhere artificial tips to the nail. Comes in many forms, including brush-on, squeeze tubes, liquids, and gels.

NAIL HARDENER: A coating placed directly on the natural nail to help nails become stronger and harder. Also referred to as nail strengthener.

NAIL HYDRATOR: A coating made of oils, soy, aloe, or other kinds of moisture to help restore moisture to dehydrated nails.

NAIL PLATE: The exposed, hard portion of the nail, composed of over 100 layers of nail cells, keratin, and other tissues.

NAIL SIDE WALLS: The fleshy areas where the nail bed and finger skin meet.

NIPPERS: A sharp tool used to trim away dead skin from the nail plate.

PARAFFIN WAX: A white, odorless, and tasteless wax used with heat as a treatment to open pores and trap moisture in the skin.

PEDICURE: Treatment to care for the feet and toenails, including soaking, moisturizing, trimming, filing, and polishing.

POLISH: A coating composed of nitrocellulose, resin, and pigment used as a cosmetic enhancement as well as to strengthen and protect nails.

POLISH REMOVER: Liquid used to break down and remove nail polish and other nail enhancements. Some removers are made of ethyl acetate and others are acetone-based.

PUMICE STONE: Used to remove dry dead skin and reduce the size of corns and calluses.

QUICK-DRY TREATMENT: A coating that speeds the drying time of wet polish, available in spray and drop formulas.

REFLEXOLOGY: The practice of massaging the hands and feet in specific areas where nerve ending are located, in order to bring relief to corresponding body parts according to reflexology maps.

RIDGE FILLER: A coating that fills the ridges and wrinkles on the nail plate, giving the nail a smoother appearance.

TOE SEPARATORS: Pieces of foam with grooves to create space between each toe to prevent smudging while polish dries.

TOP COAT: A coating made primarily of acrylic that dries to a hard finish, creating a chip-, peel-, and scratch-resistant surface.

WOODEN PUSHER: A tool used to remove excess cuticle tissue and dirt from the nail. Also referred to as an orangewood stick.

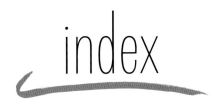

index

A

acetone, 27, 58, 64–65, 107, 136–7
acrylic paint, 113, 128–31, 144–5, 148–59, 162–3, 170–73, 176–87, 192–9, 202–203
argyle, 156–7
Art Deco, 166–7
artificial tips, 23, 32, 43, 75
angled brush, 112, 148–9, 156–7, 180–1
aromatherapy, 92–95 98, 104
autumn leaves, 188–9

B

base coat, 35–37, 41, 58, 60–63, 68–70, 80, 84, 114–213
beauty queen, 194–5
bergamot oil, 93
botanicals, 26, 70, 78, 91–92
bow, 150–1
brown sugar, 93, 95
buffer, 28, 32–33, 64–65, 68–70, 79, 86–87, 107

C

calluses, 17, 29, 70, 73, 83
camouflage, 124–5
chamomile, 92, 94, 96
chamomile and rose treatment for dry feet, 96
checkered print, 154–5
children, 65, 89
chipping, 28, 41, 79, 83
cleaning, 16, 18, 25, 33, 65, 68–69, 79, 83,
cleanser, 16, 18
clippers, 30, 33, 82, 107
corns, 17, 29
cotton, 27, 29, 64, 69, 79, 80, 82, 84, 115, 126

court jester, 202–203
crosshatch, 140–1
crystals, 52–57, 64, 134–5, 138–9, 200–201, 204–5, 212–13
crystal flowers, 100–201
cuticle, 12–13, 30–31, 42–43, 45, 58, 72–73, 74, 78–84, 86, 95–96, 118, 144, 168, 194, 206
cuticle remover, 26, 31, 65, 69, 83, 107

D

dark crystal, 204–5
detail brush, 112, 150–3, 170–3, 176–7, 180–3, 194–9
dotted frames, 114–5
dotter, 64, 112–23, 136–7, 146–53, 162–3, 172–5, 178–83, 186–91, 194–5, 208–9

E

eucalyptus, 92, 95

F

fabric, 58, 77, 128–9
fan brush, 112
feathers, 61
files, nail and foot, 13, 18, 28–29, 33, 63, 65, 68–70, 75, 78, 82–83, 85, 89, 107–8
finger bowl, 26, 69, 79, 92, 94
flat brush, 60, 112, 136–7, 162–3, 176–7, 192–3
flowers, 116–7
foot basin, 26, 70, 83, 94, 96–97
foot care, 17
foot pain, 17–19, 92

free edge, 12–14, 18, 27, 30, 32, 74–75, 78–80, 82–85
French manicure, 23, 112, 136–9, 174–5
frosted cupcake, 180–1

G

galaxy, 130–1
gel polish, 27, 33, 42–43, 55, 57
geometric shapes, 160–1
gilded city, 212–13
ginger, 92, 95
glitter, 38–39, 59–60, 77, 112, 130–1, 134–5, 138–9, 144–5, 161, 174–5, 192–3, 212–13
grapeseed oil, 92, 96
growth treatment, 37

H

hand care, 16–17
hangnail, 19, 78, 83
haute couture, 210–1
hearts, 150–1
heavy cream, 93, 95–96
honey, 93, 95–96
hygiene, 18
hyponychium, 12–13

I

infection, 18, 92
ingrown nails, 13, 19, 82, 85
invigorating hand exfoliator, 95

J

Jackson Pollock, 120–1
jojoba oil, 92–93, 95–96

L

lace, 58, 178–9
lavender, 92, 96–97